CFS

Is A

Call For Soulwork

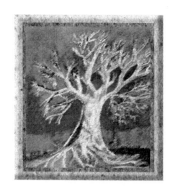

Discover the Hidden Hope of Chronic Fatigue Syndrome

Gretchen Brooks Nassar, MA

Material in Chapter 5: from ANATOMY OF THE SPIRIT by Caroline Myss, Ph.D.
© 1996 by Caroline Myss.
Used by permission of Harmony Books, a division of Random House, Inc.

Library of Congress Control Number: 2005930687

AUTHOR'S NOTE

The ideas and suggestions in this book are intended to supplement, not replace the advice of a trained medical professional. All matters regarding your health require medical supervision. Please consult with your physician before adopting any of the treatments in this book. For any questions regarding diagnosis and treatment, always check with your physician. The reader releases the author and publisher of any liability arising directly or indirectly from the use of this book.

Whenever it has felt appropriate, names have been changed.

Most CFS books refer to CFS patients as PWCs (People with Chronic Fatigue Syndrome). Here, however, the term "CFSer" will be used to denote people with CFS/CFIDS/ME.

*This book is dedicated to all CFS sufferers
and the chronically ill.
May you find hope in the darkness, a teacher in the pain,
and light along the path.*

A Note of Thanks

The following beings each contributed in their unique way to my soulwork and healing.

I extend my deepest gratitude to the man that stood by me through it all, my loving partner and best friend, Carl, without whom I cannot imagine my life nor what my healing journey would have looked like. Carlos, thank you for all of it.

To Sage and Rita, my "sunshines"—consistent and loving each moment of each CFS-laden day, I will always love you. To Sylvan and Sumu, thank you "twos" for brightening my every day.

To Mona, Teta, and Cecile: thank you all for your loving kindness and sincere interest in my well-being.

For constant financial support during CFS, Dad, I thank you for your generosity and love.

I owe much of my healing success to the healers/doctors who not only helped me identify the source of my symptoms, but also made excellent treatment suggestions. These healers gave me hope when others wouldn't, respected my insights regarding my body, and were the best empathetic listeners—My thanks to Jackie Fields, Michael Sutton, Oliver Pijoan, Peg Nelson, and Kay Kimball.

To my first spiritual teacher and healer, Andrew Shier, who not only helped me heal my endocrine system, but introduced me to divinity through the healing art, attunement. Thank you for the abundant support and your belief in my abilities.

Another key spiritual teacher in my life has been Neale Donald Walsch. Through the daring, inspirational messages in *Conversations With God*, my life has been forever changed. Thank you, Neale.

Deep gratitude goes out to the first editor and typist of this book, Sarita, and my special friend, Brenda, whose dedication to my manuscript enabled me to publish.

My healing journey would never have been complete without the countless books that provided answers to the CFS mystery. I thank the many authors for their CFS books.

A special thank you to author, John Robbins, author of *Diet for a New America* whose book led me to make the soulful change to vegetarian. Thank you for your courage in exposing the truth about the agribusiness as well as your efforts to free billions of animals from a life of misery, premature death, and abuse. I thank all people involved in work dedicated to giving animals a voice, rights, and love.

I want to thank Oprah for your inspiring show that offered me much needed catharsis, connection, and inspiration during times in the depths of CFS isolation. I applaud you for your dedication to heal the planet.

Finally, it has meant so much whenever people have declared their belief in me. Thank you Mom for that. And thank you Lara, Mona, and Carlos.

To the many readers: thank you for your insights and helpful feedback.

For my healing and the creation of this book, thank you spirit of it all, thank you God.

TABLE OF CONTENTS

DEAR READER

Today is February 12, 2004. The very first time I heard of CFS was when I picked up Susan Lark's CFS book in 1994. I was a student at Antioch Graduate School in Keene, NH, and I was on the path to becoming a psychotherapist. I was also beginning to meet CFS head on. In my car, when I studied, and every morning I experienced symptoms of paralyzing fatigue, inability to focus or concentrate, and throat-clogging morning mucous—all leading me to the CFS bookshelves in a local bookshop.

I am not sure how I knew where to look, but like so many other times in my life, the right book found me, just as CFS had. This year marked the beginning of my CFS journey.

Just as I had done so many times that fateful year and the several that followed, today I once again ponder CFS, read about it, and still wonder: "Do I have CFS?" Conversely, throughout most of this past year, I felt done with the disease, often explaining when people asked, "How is your health?" that I felt I was over the chronic fatigue, yet still healing some of the related imbalances.

Today, however, I debate whether I am truly over CFS. Much to my dismay, this past November, the old sluggish, "moving through quicksand" feeling returned. A naturopath suggested it could be my thyroid. *How could this be?* I protested. It couldn't be true, not after years of investigation, blood tests, thyroid meds, and finally elimination of those same meds and a return to energy-filled days (confirmed by a normal thyroid test). Had I slid back somehow? It couldn't be. It can't be.

Today, I don't yet know what is going on, what brought that wasteland fatigue back, but I suspect it is at the least related to my thyroid. Waves of sadness, frustration, and anger wash over me. Then, the tide recedes and I return calm, focused yet again on my healing.

Is my CFS over? Is it ever over? As you move through the pages of my CFS journey, my *Call For Soulwork*, you will discover apparent contradictions. You will hear tales of hope, words of inspiration, and then other times the suffocating sadness and bleakness of CFS will emerge. Both will be real; both are. CFS and its *call* are full of the dark and the light. But mostly, this book expands on the light side and helps you see how even amidst the darkness of CFS' most sobering symptoms, you can feel hopeful, you can trust life, and yourself.

Between 1997 and 2000, my days were filled with CFS. Most days were lonely self-discovery sessions focused on reading, investigating, trying healing remedies, and writing. Initially this book came to me as an un-welcomed guest every morning around 3 a.m. For two years this is how it went: first a chapter title would declare itself in my mind, then the chapter would follow flowing from my hand to pad of paper. I made no attempt to contemplate the words, their meanings and message; I simple wrote what came, and *Call For Soulwork* thus emerged.

In 2000, the first draft of this book (filling two journals) was complete and handed over to an editor. She and I worked together for several months then stopped. I was too overwhelmed by the enormity of work required to refine the draft into a finished product. The book was shelved and temporarily forgotten.

Three years later, after having completed my master's degree and having reached a crossroads in my business as private ESL instructor, I was brought back to the book. Like the early morning muse of years prior, inspiration returned and I knew I was ready to finish the editing process. I couldn't bear the thought of leaving the book to never see the light of another person's eyes. I knew that *Call* was not intended exclusively for me. It needed readers, people who might find wisdom in its pages.

So here I am, and here you are. You are the reader that *Call For Soulwork* was meant for; perhaps you are someone whose life has been forever uprooted by the uninvited guest, CFS. Perhaps you are in need of support, hope, and ideas, and you need to hear from someone like yourself; someone who knows CFS from the inside and understands that the chronic fatigue that you are experiencing is not for naught. You deserve to know that. We all do.

I truly hope that *Call For Soulwork* gives you the strength to stand up and declare that you are not CFS' victim, nor is CFS your perpetrator. This is not an easy road you have embarked on. It is not what you envisioned for your life. Neither is it what I planned for my own. Nevertheless, here we find CFS in our lives.

Please understand that CFS is not just an illness, nor an enemy. To see how CFS can be your teacher, your *Call For Soulwork*, read on. Underlying the *Call* is this message: *healing CFS is a divine journey, for within it, one sees, tastes, and lives in the darkness, yet paradoxically is embraced by the light.* As you read, you will discover what it means to experience the blessings of CFS.

May your CFS become your most amazing journey, your most life-enhancing *Call For Soulwork*. May you feel, through the healing process, in every moment of every hour and through every symptom, that you are indeed healing.

Bless you, and bless your healing journey.

CFS sufferer, CFS survivor, CFS victor,

Gretchen

A Note About Call's Format

This book, though divinely inspired, is also CFS inspired. That is, CFS caused this book to be, as did divinity. Had it not been for CFS, I would not have written this. And, had it not been for my wee-morning muse awakening me abruptly on so many a night, this book would never have transpired.

As part of any CFS journey, we must find our own way. In keeping with that, feel free to read this book in any way that works for you. It is not necessary that you read every page or chapter, nor that you read this in a linear fashion. What is most important is that you find a reading approach best suited to you and your journey.

I have had numerous opportunities to try and read as a CFSer—many of my efforts, unfortunately thwarted. My many reading attempts often have been met with word-dances (where I could not focus and the words jumped around on the page) or times the text would enter my mind, only to immediately go back out again. Consequently, I have learned what worked and didn't for my CFS-compromised mind.

This book is designed with such a CFSer in mind. The font style and size, the page layout, and even the repetition of ideas are by no accident, but rather an attempt to aid the mentally clouded CFS sufferer.

I hope that these elements help you absorb what is here. In addition to the elements above, "chapter gems" (key ideas in each chapter) have been repeated for you at the end of each chapter for easy end-of-the-chapter reviews or later retrieval. I hope that all of these factors enhance your reading experience, facilitate your understanding, and refresh your memory.

CFS

Is A

Call For Soulwork

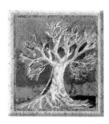

Discover the Hidden Hope
of Chronic Fatigue Syndrome

Gretchen Brooks Nassar, MA

CFS Fact Sheet

CFS, also referred to as CFIDS (Chronic Fatigue Immune Deficiency Syndrome), is a legitimate disease/syndrome.

It typically affects every bodily system: neurological (mind) immunological (immune system), hormonal, gastrointestinal (digestion), and musculoskeletal (muscles).

CFS is not simply the experience of extreme fatigue; it is an illness/syndrome manifesting through hundreds of symptoms.

It is a serious, life-altering, chronic (long-term) condition, not only impacting a person's body, but also their mind and spirit.

There are approximately 800,000 CFS cases in America today.

CFS is three times more prevalent in women than men and it impacts every race.

It is primarily an adult disease afflicting 20-40 year olds.

As of 2004, the medical establishment has yet to identify the causes of CFS, lacks a CFS diagnostic test, and has been unable to identify a cure/cures; however researchers are working to change these facts.

To be diagnosed with CFS, you must show at least 4 of these symptoms:
1. *a life-altering fatigue lasting six months or longer*
2. *impaired memory and mental concentration*
3. *sore throat*
4. *joint pain*
5. *sleep disturbances*
6. *atypical headaches*
7. *post-exertion (exercise) exhaustion*

CALL FOR SOULWORK CHECKLIST

Most of you will invariably see CFS as an illness to be cured from the outside-in. You will visit doctors who will tell you what to do about what, the outside. You will look at your plight as a physical one to be addressed from the outside. I am going to suggest to you that CFS is more than a disease of the physical, the body. CFS certainly lives in the cells, but also dwells in the mind, and the heart.

I am going to suggest to you that you not only do things to help your body heal the sickness but also help your mind, and your soul. This is what holistic means: body, mind, and soul.

CFS is a holistic illness that best heals when dealt with holistically. I say this not from what I've read on the subject (and I've read a lot), but rather from my own personal experience. Ultimately it is our experience and our knowing that leads us. Let your own knowing, that which comes from your heart, guide you in whatever treatments and healing modalities you try. Trust yourself first. Trust your body and your experience, not someone else's.

There is no limit to what you can do to heal. Many books speak to this. Most of them tackle the healing from the outside-in. *Heal the symptoms*, they say. *Heal the body;* I say. Heal more than your body; heal your body, mind, and soul. Where and how you begin is not important. Just that you begin, is. Here, I am giving you a list to consider. Hopefully, you can use this list as an aid to healing yourself holistically. It is not the cure. No *one* thing is. CFS is healed when many imbalances are healed, imbalances of the body, mind, and soul.

So be well and go forth in whatever way you know is right for you.

THE CHECKLIST

Here is a list to help you look at CFS holistically, and to help you identify what's important to your healing process.

PHYSICAL

I have ruled-out, checked out, or treated:

Candida Albicans (yeast syndrome)

Allergies

Thyroid imbalance

Hormonal imbalance: estrogen, progesterone,
    testosterone, and DHEA

Sugar metabolism: Hypoglycemia, Syndrome X, Diabetes

Nutritional deficiencies (i.e., B vitamins, magnesium)

Sleep disturbances

Diet: How is my diet? Does it feed my body and my soul?

Do I get regular exercise?

Do I spend time enjoying nature: light, air, water and soil?

Do I experience beauty in my life?

MENTAL

Am I able to concentrate? Are my short and
long-term memories disturbed?

Do I challenge myself mentally?

Do I use my mind regularly?

Am I conscious of my thinking patterns?

Do I believe in myself?

What are my typical mental messages?

How do I think about my life and my CFS?

Is my mind reeling or stressed?

What can I do to calm and focus my mind?

Do I think of myself as an empowered person or victim?

EMOTIONAL

Do I like myself?

How do I feel about my life?

Is joy a big part of my life? Do I wish it to be?

How do I feel about CFS?

How do I express my feelings? Do I express them?

What are my feelings regarding my daily life:
home, work, and relationships?

Do I feel stressed?

What can I do to feel less stressed?

SPIRITUAL

What is the meaning of life?

What is the meaning of *my* life?

Who am I?

Why am I here?

Do I connect to a higher source, spirit, the Divine?

Do I engage in spiritual practice, ritual?

Do I see life as a gift?

Do I feel or experience the Divine spirit in my life?

Am I creative? Would creativity serve my soul?

What does my soul yearn for? (What is missing?)

RELATIONSHIPS

Are relationships important to me?

How are my relationships?

Do I have any unfinished business with others?

Can I trust others? Do I feel supported emotionally
    by others?

Do I have positive relationships with co-workers,
    friends, neighbors, and family?

Who are my trusted confidants?

ENVIRONMENT

Have I been exposed to any toxins that may have impacted
my health (at work, in the home, in the air, water or soil)?

Have I eaten or taken something that my body may have
had adverse reactions to?

Do I get outside regularly?

Are my home and workplace sources of peace or stress?

SOULWORK

Do I strive to improve myself?

Do I ask myself what I want from life? Do I work towards it?

Do I treat myself well?

Do I deserve better?

What is my pace in life? Am I too fast to enjoy what's
right before me?

Do I experience "lack" in: time, money, love, freedom,
or _____?

Do I give myself free time?

Do I have fun?

PHYSICAL HEALING

Could I benefit from any of the following:

Vitamin/nutritional supplements

Colon cleanses

Dietary changes

Massage

Spa treatments

Yoga

Meditation

Visualization

Prayer

Energy work

Homeopathy

Aromatherapy

Herbology

Naturopathy

Ayurvedic Medicine

Chinese medicine

Cranio-sacral work

Psychotherapy/Coaching

Spiritual retreats

Chiropractic

Nature experience

Dance/singing/writing/art

Entertainment: theater, movies, restaurants

Humor

A Cry for Validation

I Cry for Validation,
Please,
I just need validation
Agree with me, damn it!
I'm not okay
can't you see what's happening?
Mucous in mouth, white-coated tongue,
sleepless, wakeful nights...
None of this is alarming?

You notice nearly none of it.
questioning my motives
for illness—
Like CFS is some kind of criminal behavior
But it's an invisible crime.

I sleep weird hours: no work, no routine
What you see are behavioral
oddities, and not the facts of my physical and
        emotional changes.

You judge me
I am wrong not to work,

CFS, a mere excuse
Well, Ex—cuse me!
No one chooses illness
Well...not consciously.
My illness is real, physical
an uncomfortable, uninvited entity.

Yes, I am befriending it.
Yes, CFS has changed my life.
I let it in now and it's not my enemy
Sometimes I pretend it isn't a part of me, but
CFS and I are real!
Can't you see?
It's validation I seek;
I'm not crazy.

Internally
strange molecules dance,
and destroy
my brain and emotions
I feel temporarily invaded.

Inexplicable rage; crazed
lady
lost in a parking lot;
dizzy disorientation.
Here I am seemingly overpowered
by miniscule chemicals,

but you don't see them,
only I feel them.
Trust me, I know what I am
feeling.
Trust me,
Am I crazy?
Trust the raging banshee?
You don't see much,
not
even my struggles with disorientation, panic and
debilitating fatigue.

You don't see me; only your memories, only your
 skewed perceptions of my reality are what you see.

Validation;
I need to be heard.
Validation;
I need to be understood.
I need to have someone say:
"Yes your feelings are real, your symptoms
     are physiological
phenomena.
Yes, you have CFS;
I'm sorry you have CFS.
Can I help?
You have CFS,
What's that like?"

Validation
takes the past pain of your judgment and denial—
    all away.

I can forgive you.
I do forgive you.
You are blind, afraid to open your eyes to the truth.
Denial frees you from responsibility, from feeling the
    need to do anything.

You are free to judge.
I'll find my peace, and I'll find others who believe in me,
and the reality of
my disease.

I'll find my peace.

1
INTRODUCTION

After I had been sick for several months, it became clear to me that I was changing in fundamental ways and that I would never go back to my "old self." One day, when I was taking my morning walk across the mesa, I heard myself muttering under my breath, over and over like a droning chant, "I don't know who I am anymore. I don't know who I am anymore." Like many sick people, I had begun to realize that my illness was not so much a state of being as a process of transformation."

Kat Duff, author of CFS Book: *The Alchemy of Illness*

I used to wake up every morning around three a.m. and feel wide-awake and mentally alert, but physically light—as if I had no body. At such times, words would spin out of control in my mind. From the moment I broke slumber, words formed chapter titles and told the story of what CFS was all about—not the ugly story, not the story of painful symptoms and unwanted experiences, but a story of hope, meaning, and of *being* with Chronic Fatigue Syndrome. At the time, I didn't know I was writing a book. I just knew that when I wrote the words and ideas that were swimming in my mind, they made sense; they made sense out of what didn't: an illness that I didn't want.

The words taught me that I could live happily with

CFS. I could learn to *be* with and accept my illness. I didn't have to fight to heal. Healing, I discovered, came from acceptance and seeing what a blessing CFS was. The words flowed effortlessly from my mind onto paper. I'd write furiously. Energy that I hadn't experienced since the onset of my CFS, strangely came through my mind, out my hand—channeling my thoughts to paper. I had begun to heal. As I wrote, I healed and learned what it meant to have CFS; I learnt how to transform my tragedy.

Admittedly, there were those times when I'd awaken in the middle of the night and not grab my pen and journal. Instead, I simply lay there, with a relaxed body but my mind racing. I lived in my mind. Everything that I couldn't do physically was replaced by what I could do in my mind. In my mind, I accomplished everyday activities: cleaning house, doing laundry, calling friends, and more extraordinary activities like writing a book and teaching inspiring classes. Later in the day, usually about noon (after being awake for hours), I would grow exhausted and unable to focus. Everything turned to haze: my mind, thoughts, and vision. I could focus on nothing. The fatigue that had eluded me in the middle of the night, now dragged me back to bed or the couch. Hating it, I would try to stay awake, sometimes drinking a coffee, other times forcing myself to walk, or to clean. More often than not, I'd give in and go back to bed. Later, when waking up from my mid-day nap, everything that had felt so good, so meaningful in the middle of the night, had vanished. I felt groggy, lethargic, and depressed.

My prior motivation to write chapter after chapter was now replaced by a feeling of absolute disdain, disdain for how I felt and for how I saw myself: a worthless dough-girl.

I've lived with CFS for the past ten years. In that time, I've left everything I once knew behind: who I was; what I wanted for myself; and what was important to me—my prior life vanished.

But over the span of ten years, CFS became not just a life-altering illness in the negative sense, but a positive, life-inspiring experience. Just how this happened is still somewhat a mystery to me. Though CFS enveloped my body with symptom after symptom, the most meaningful CFS changes were those visiting my mind and taking root deep in my soul. Over time, I made choices that helped me gain power over an illness that seemed to disempower. I decided to do three things that would lay the foundation to seeing chronic fatigue syndrome as more than just an undesirable illness, but as a *Call For Soulwork*. These were: 1) accept all that CFS brings; 2) do everything I can to heal, while simultaneously not requiring healing in order to value myself or my life; and 3) trust that CFS had something great to offer me.

There are many great books on the subject of CFS (refer to CFS Resources), many which emphasize the physiological nature of CFS (while also providing healing alternatives). Some offer suggestions about how to live with CFS. Few, however, present the view of CFS as anything more than an illness to overcome. Few provide tools and ideas for how to better live emotionally/spiritually with your CFS. Few refer to your healing as a process or to its holistic nature, even though CFS encompasses body, mind, and spirit, and healing CFS entails a journey of body, mind, and spirit.

Call For Soulwork shows you how CFS is so much more than an illness that has disrupted and altered your entire life. This book is not intended to be a "how to" in the traditional sense. I cannot provide you with the magical treatment that will suddenly return your life to pre-CFS. Only you, with the help of others, can discover the specific requirements for your healing.

I am here to help you in a different way. A *Call For Soulwork* is a new type of "how to" book. Rather than instructing you on "how to heal," this book teaches "how to BE" with your CFS in new transformational ways. When you learn to see CFS as your teacher, your experience of CFS changes from that of battleground to one of relationship. In relationship with CFS, you will see that this illness can help you look at yourself and your life in new ways.

In the book *Tuesdays with Morrie*, the author Mitch Albom tells us that our culture does not teach us to value ourselves. I agree. When I consider what our society values, I hear, "Work hard, present yourself as professional and attractive, and get everything you can: a home, a beautiful car, and the latest technology." The focus is on the material things of life, the externals. These are the things that are supposed to bring about our happiness. Anyone who has chased after these things sooner or later discovers the painful and important truth. Money, beauty, and work will not provide happiness. Not even health can guarantee it. Happiness, like health, is something you cannot buy. It is something that cannot come from outside of yourself. Happiness and health must be created from within.

We are taught day in and day out through the media, in schools, and in the workplace, that everything that matters is external to us. Our value lies outside, on the surface: in our appearance, through our job titles, in our material possessions. CFS teaches differently. You do not have to have anything, not even health, to be of value. You do not have to "do" anything, either. Societal messages about accomplishment through work and possessions and appearances are simply that, messages. *Not all messages are truth.*

Here is a message from nature. Everyday my loving cat Sage relaxed the day away doing absolutely nothing. But was she value-less? I cannot imagine what my life would have been without this incredible being. Her loving presence was always with me with never a negative word, only a reassuring purr. Sage's value is hardly recognized by the societal myths described here, but her value in my life is undeniable.

Call For Soulwork is not going to emphasize what you can take, do, or try in order to heal. More healing techniques are found in other fine CFS books. This book is going to help you in a new way. It's going to empower you to see CFS as your teacher. It's going to show you several ways to view and experience your illness.

When you begin to embrace your CFS as a benevolent teacher, you begin to heal. This book will help you value yourself and your experiences throughout your healing journey. The principles I share here have helped me and I am confident they can help you, too. I know that these words, which I spent many sleepless nights writing and many lethargic days rewriting, are not just for me; they are for you, too.

GEMS

To experience CFS as a Call For Soulwork:

Accept all that CFS brings; do everything you can to heal, while simultaneously not requiring healing in order to value your self or life, and trust CFS has something great to offer.

You do not have to have anything, not even health, to be of value. You do not have to 'do' anything either.

2
THE CFS TREE

It may be that when we no longer know what to do, we have come to our real work and that when we no longer know which way to go, we have begun our real journey.

Wendell Berry

Over the past ten years since living with CFS, I've devoured many books: books on CFS, books on healing, books explaining Candida, books about herbs, nutrition, aromatherapy, energy, and the chakras. I've tried countless treatments and met with MD's, ND's, acupuncturists, herbalists, nutritionists, ayurvedic practitioners, energy-healers, homeopaths, and massage therapists. I've practiced self-body massage, yoga, attunement, visualization, and journaling. I've attended workshops and facilitated them. I've expressed my soul through creativity: photography, drawing, tarot, writing articles, and now, this book. My healing journey has taken me through the physical to the emotional, mental, and spiritual aspects of my life.

There are many who have struggled and continue to struggle to find what heals or cures CFS. I too, at times have taken this approach, only to eventually discover that

Chronic Fatigue Syndrome is not something to eradicate with a treatment weapon. Rather, it is a teacher and guide for living. CFS is not simply about the unpleasant and unwanted. Its power in our lives is so vast and wide that it wreaks havoc on our bodies, minds, and emotions, yet its true purpose is to bring about change.

At first, the changes are resisted and resented. We hate CFS for its myriad symptoms, for its disruption of our lives. Energy and vitality are seemingly sucked out from us. We grow angry, depressed, and listless. CFS changes us, and at first, it's nothing but ugly. Later, as we let go of our resistance and let go of our dark, depressed feelings, we open ourselves to CFS' presence. We discover over time, through trust, patience, and exploration, that CFS is our teacher. CFS is a strong, ever-present tree whose presence and growth astounds and disturbs those of us who have it, and the medical doctors who don't understand it.

CFS is not simply a virus, bug, or microorganism thriving on a weakened system. No, CFS does not exist solely in the physical reality we all see. CFS has roots in the invisible world as well. CFS manifestations not only shutdown many of your physical capabilities: giving you weakness, fatigue beyond belief, headaches and pain, but it also alters your mind from intelligent to unintelligible. CFS robs you of your body, your mind, and your sense of self—the person you thought you were before its invasion. By all accounts, CFS appears to be an enemy that has literally invaded your world on every level—physical, mental, emotional, and

22

spiritual. Many people try to understand and find treatments for the physical symptoms of CFS. However, this approach fails to recognize CFS in its entirety. CFS is far more than a physical illness. CFS is a *Call For Soulwork!*

CFS wants you to take the *Call.* When you do, you change yourself in ways that make you strong, stronger than before. The *Call* asks you to alter your lifestyle, redirect your vision, uproot your memories, and walk a new path. If CFS were simply about physical health, then *why would it profoundly alter every aspect of our lives? Why rob us of everything, if only to be reckoned with physically?*

There is a lot more we can do with CFS in addition to treating the physical symptoms. Our healing journey begins when we hear the *Call* and recognize that there is something in our lives, something about ourselves that would benefit from a change. CFS helps us to identify what needs to change.

My *Call For Soulwork* began the day I could no longer drive without falling asleep at the wheel. My *call* continued as I lost my ability to concentrate while reading. When, after sleeping twelve hours each night awakening to chokes on sour phlegm and sluggishness that would not quit, I knew something was off.

Sure, I was depressed. After all, I hated the brutality of the northeast weather and missed friends, family, and the California sun. But something else was wrong, too. And I didn't understand it. I just noticed *it* and kept on noticing *it*

23

until *it* became so powerful in my life that I had no choice but to let *it* become my life. *It* drove me to leave graduate school and who I thought I was, behind. First, however, I would drive across country with Carl and my cats for yet a third time to transfer to another Antioch campus (the second one in two years). Soon, I would have to leave that school, too, dropping everything.

It was then in 1995 that CFS became my life. Except for planning Carl's and my wedding, there were no commitments, school, or work. I simply couldn't do much of anything. *It* wouldn't let me. *It* had taken over. *It* was CFS. That is how my *Call For Soulwork* journey began.

That year, I turned my life over to CFS and decided that I would learn from it, that I would do everything I could to heal. That was the beginning of my journey toward healing.

That summer, in the beautiful warmth of the Santa Barbara sun, I began my healing journey by learning a new way of life; a life all about *being*, not *doing*. My version of *being* began with simply sitting still in my favorite pink chair, soaking up the comfort and warmth of the sun's rays. I began to relax, and listen to what my body had to say.

Despite all the beauty surrounding me, deep within I was alone and lonely. For the second time in my life, I had moved hundreds of miles from my family, and this time, I had also moved far away from my primary support person and fiance, Carl. With no family and few friends around except for the presence of my faithful, ever loving cat-companions,

I was very much alone, and I began to focus all my energy on my healing journey with CFS.

The more time I spent hanging out with my CFS, the more I realized hidden meaning lay beneath the pain and misery. I had yet to understand the teachings, but I knew there was unearthing to do—profound, deep learning. I was ready.

More recently, I've come to appreciate CFS as my teacher—my *Call For Soulwork*. I've come to envision CFS not simply as an illness, but as my own special *tree* full of life and beauty. The *Call* asks us to envision CFS as a tree and to unearth the mystery beneath our CFS and see the beautiful tree that grew for us to lean against and learn from. CFS teaches us its presence is not simply a menace to destroy. Eventually, the time will come when we will no longer need the tree. We'll unearth its roots and the tree will topple, returning to the soil from which it was born.

When you envision CFS as a tree, you begin to understand its complexity and the interconnectedness between all of its parts. Pondering the growth of each root and branch, one from another, helps us to discover and understand our unique CFS mystery.

CFS is not a dark, inexplicable illness we must conquer; CFS is an incredible, life-changing tree. Before it grew, CFS was invisible to you, deep beneath the soil of your awareness. It took root in a rich, dark, fertile soil consisting of a mixture of your past: your thoughts and attitudes, life events, stressors, emotional issues, diet, and lifestyle choices. All of these together created a fertile soil from which your CFS tree could grow. Over time, your CFS tree developed strong roots and grew from the invisible, from beneath the soil, to eventually become visible in your life. Symptoms appeared, sprouting from the soil of your past—strange, daunting fatigue, and flu-like symptoms. At first, you suffered, but then shrugged them off, believing those symptoms were a passing thing. You didn't realize their power and you did not realize that you had just met the sprouts of what would grow into a very large tree.

As time passed, the CFS trunk (fed by the rich soil of your past) developed branches large and small. Branches began to appear as recognizable symptoms and illness—and you began to resist. Little did you know, you were growing a very strong tree, a tree that would take over your entire life.

The first branches to sprout from the CFS trunk were big and strong and took advantage of your body's already weakened immune, nervous, and endocrine systems. These *large branches* presented themselves as other *illnesses*: hypoglycemia, candida, and hypothyroidism, for example. From the larger branches of illness grew *smaller*, intertwining branches: the *symptoms*. The symptoms were both pervasive and subtle: the endless fatigue, mind-fog, headaches, painful joints, and abdominal problems.

In a short time, you experienced the full-fledged presence of the CFS tree. Each symptom, represented by a small branch, extends from yet a larger branch: a larger, more pervasive symptom. And that larger branch, in turn, grows from an even bigger branch or illness. Each large branch represents a condition/illness (candida) while smaller ones symbolize your day to day symptoms.

With every branch, symptom, and ailment, your experience emerges from the trunk: your CFS. As your little branches of painful, unwanted symptoms crowd your awareness, the trunk disappears under a canopy of interwoven, thick and thin branches. And what seems to be an experience filled with daunting ailments and annoying little symptoms, is in fact a life filled with the presence of a huge CFS tree.

Caught up in days of misery entangled in your branches, you can only think about one thing: chopping down your CFS tree. "Leave CFS forever behind!" you fantasize. But your tree stands tall, strong, and resilient because its roots are well grounded and well nourished by you, its keeper.

Despite the CFS tree's incredible beauty, nobody— not you, not anyone—can see anything beyond the nuisance. The tree is an unwelcome visitor in your garden, and no one seems to be able to chop it down. Despite your search here and there for the strongest, most powerful tree-chopper, the only people you encounter are tree-trimmers, and they only trim away one or two branches at a time, leaving behind an intact CFS tree. So, you thank your doctor, homeopath, ND, or whomever it was who helped you to eliminate one symptom (one little-bitty branch from your enormous tree), and you remain overwhelmed, angry, and frustrated because you can't see any part of your tree as pretty or purposeful.

You cannot see the shade that your tree provides on sun-baked days. You are blinded to the haven your tree provides for the local squirrels and birds. All you see is a menace, a tree that has uprooted your backyard, your garden—your life!

If you want, CFS can be the most menacing of trees crowding out every inch of your life. Or, it can be an awesome teacher whose little branches, though tedious and unpleasant, don't prevent bright, sunny rays of hope from shining in. You can choose to continue viewing your tree as something you plan to chop down with the best, most powerful tree-chopping remedy. Or, you can look closely at your tree and examine the relationship between its web of branches, trunk, and roots. You can dig in the soil of your life—the painful thoughts, unresolved issues, disturbing events, and uncomfortable experiences—soil that nourished the development of the very roots of your CFS tree. And you can decide to nourish your tree no more.

Once you let go of the need to chop your CFS tree down, you free yourself to explore the tree beyond its physical symptoms: its branches and huge trunk. You can probe it's dark recesses where the roots grow and unearth what's there. When you unearth the roots, the tree can no longer survive. On the other hand, when you attempt to cut it down, ignoring the roots, you leave behind the impetus for birth of some other kind of tree; if not CFS, then something else, but nevertheless, something unwanted.

Each CFS tree looks, feels, and is unique. Each has its own branch configuration and its own unique roots of thoughts and feelings. I cannot unearth your tree, nor can any doctor, or healing practitioner—only you can do your own healing. Only you know the soil of your life experiences—your illness branches, and your symptoms. And only you can learn to value all that your tree has to teach you. The rest of us: your friends, family, doctors, and myself, can offer our thoughts, help and wisdom, but it is *you* who must do the healing work. We can also suggest treatments, but ultimately, it is *you* who decides what actions to take. *You* decide what to do, what to think and how to live. *You* decide whether to swing from your CFS branches, sit against its trunk, or dive deep into its dark, rich soil.

Please join me as I unearth my own CFS tree. In so doing, I hope that you, too, will discover how to unearth your own tree and act on your CFS as a *Call For Soulwork*. It's time to see the beauty in your tree's adversity. Our CFS trees have the power to uproot our lives as we know them, but they also have the power to provide the atmosphere for new understanding, new perspectives and ways of *being* with our illness, and with ourselves.

The CFS tree is our *Call For Soulwork*—the *call* to look beyond the tree and find what it will take to create a new, healthier you.

GEMS

The CFS Tree:

CFS took root in rich, dark fertile soil consisting of your past: your thoughts and attitudes, life events, stressors, emotional issues, diet, and lifestyle choices.

You can choose to continue viewing your tree as something you plan to chop down with the best, most powerful tree chopping remedy. Or, you can look closely at your tree and understand the relationship between its web of branches, trunk, and roots.

Our CFS trees have the power to uproot our lives as we know them, and they have the power to provide new understanding, perspectives, and ways of being with our illness.

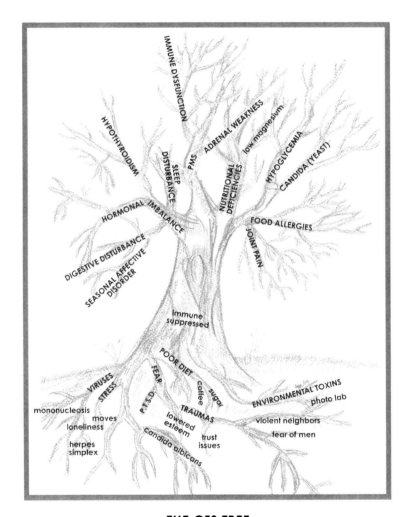

THE CFS TREE

3

To You, My CFS Friend

To heal is to touch with love that which we previously touched with fear.

Stephen Levine

You have come to this book seeking answers. Just as you sought out this book, CFS sought you out and is your messenger. CFS has come to awaken you to more of yourself. CFS is a blessed presence and cursed shadow. Until now, you have probably only known the dark-side: your symptoms, the chronic exhaustion, malaise, and pain. Now, I would like to acquaint you with the lighter side of CFS. It has more to give than unwanted symptoms.

If CFS' only purpose were to cause us pain and unhappiness, then doctors would find a cure, and we'd all reach for it and have CFS no more. But doctors don't have a cure; or have they found a clear-cut cause. The reason behind this is CFS is not simply a physical malady requiring a physical cure, no! CFS is more, much more, and it is up to you to discover what that "more" is.

CFS strikes nearly a million Americans, yet despite our many common symptoms and ailments, no two CFS experiences are exactly alike—and neither are the underlying causes. CFS is not a simple illness. Why? Its causes are too vast, its treatments too numerous. So, what are the answers? That's where you come in. That's where this book comes in.

Our health is multifaceted; it depends on well-balanced minds, emotions, and bodies. The opposite can be said of CFS. It depends on imbalanced minds, emotions, and bodies. Healing CFS involves more than finding the perfect treatment for a physical problem; it involves healing via a journey of the self. On this journey, you encounter yourself and your CFS in all its' dimensions. You are a physical, mental, emotional, and spiritual being, and your healing lies in addressing most, if not all, of these aspects of your self.

CFS as a *Call For Soulwork* insists that your illness is not merely a curse, but the strangest of blessings. It gives you a chance to focus on yourself. This is *your* time. You deserve to be happy, and you can be happy even while experiencing CFS. You no longer have to see your illness as something to deny, hide, or fight against. You can accept and embrace your CFS while simultaneously discovering it has much more to offer than its symptoms and discomfort.

To you, my CFS friends I wish great discovery, transformative insights, and abundant healing.

GEMS

CFS is not just a physical malady requiring a physical cure; it is much more—it is up to you to discover what the "more" is.

Healing CFS involves more than finding the per-fect treatment for a physical problem; it involves healing via a journey of the self.

4

To Friends and Family

All that I give, I give to myself.

Gerald Jampolsky

Cfs is an elusive, invisible illness that has remained hidden in the closet for too long. People with chronic fatigue are not acknowledged, or adequately understood by society. Our society, yours and mine, is hung up on wellness; hung up on *doing*. For most of us, excellent health is the only acceptable state. It is deified in our society, because without it, you are unable to *do*, and in a *doing* society like ours, *doing* is everything.

Chronic Fatigue Syndrome, in many ways, is about learning to *BE*. It's about learning to love who you are without having to *do* anything. Chronic fatigue is the antithesis to what our society idolizes: *do, do, do*.

In such a *doing* world, you: parents, siblings, and friends of the CFSer, can give the CFSer the gift that society does not—the gift of your acceptance and love. Accept the CFSer who cannot *do*. Give your acceptance to the CFS sufferer who cannot participate in so much of what everyone deems normal. Love this person for who she is, not for what she once did, or who she appeared to be as a professional, or in her role as mother, sister, daughter, whomever. Beneath the layers of activities and roles, there is a person for you to discover, to know, or get to know.

Chronic fatigue feels lousy and appears not to make sense. It robs us of our soul while paradoxically giving us a unique opportunity to uncover, discover, and create ourselves in new and exciting ways. Truthfully, the physiological aspects of CFS strip us of our vitality, and the very nature of this illness erodes our sense of self and robs us of everything. And ultimately—after we've passed through the dark tunnel of our journey of pain, suffering, and loss—CFS helps us to reencounter and redefine ourselves in beautiful, new ways.

First, we must lose the very person we thought ourselves to be, only later to walk the path of our true self: the person beneath the roles, beneath the appearances, and beneath previously held beliefs.

It's no coincidence that CFS frequently happens to achievers, super-achievers, and doers. And it happens to shatter our whole self-concept and identity. CFS changes us. It changes who we are, who we want to become, and our world-view. CFS rearranges our priorities. What *once* mattered most, now becomes irrelevant or less important while journeying through CFS. What was once our identity is no longer because it can be no longer—not with CFS.

Everything changes with CFS, including our relationships and our relationships with you: our friends and family. When you, friends and family to a CFSer, are unable to grasp the impact of CFS—the fact that things have really changed for us—then you miss the gift that CFS has to offer you. Because disguised as it is, CFS is a gift for all who encounter it.

You: the friend, mother, brother, or the lover of the CFS sufferer, are very important to the CFSer. Through your support, love and caring, you can make what might otherwise be a lonely, bitter, and frightening journey, instead an experience that supports discovery and creation.

The CFS journey requires that the old exterior self die, and as it dies, a new self can be born. Birthing is much easier when there are supportive family members around to help out. You can help. Be the love and acceptance that the CFS sufferer yearns to experience.

Self-help Author Gerald Jampolsky, author of *Love is Letting Go of Fear*, teaches us that when you give to yourself you give to another, and when you give to another, you give to yourself. Giving doesn't mean that you give up your own life or self to care for your loved one. It simply means that you are present some of the time for your CFS friend or family member and you give him/her the compassionate side of who you are. So give of yourself, and give to yourself. For whenever you give to another, you give to yourself.

Know, too, that this is a time when the CFSer cannot give to you what she once did. This is a time for herself, her healing, and for her learning. Give respect, support, and try to understand. She is lucky to have you in her life. Your support will be helpful on her healing journey. Thank you.

GEMS

---

*People with chronic fatigue are not acknowl-
edged, nor adequately understood by society
because society is hung up on wellness and
"doing." Chronic Fatigue Syndrome is about
learning to be; learning to love who you are
without having to do anything.*

*CFS shatters our whole self-concept and identity.
CFS changes us. It changes who we are, who we
want to become, and it changes our world-view.*

5
POSSIBLE CFS ROOTS:
THE ENERGETIC BODY

You may think of this energy as flowing into us from the universe, from God, or from the Tao, but as it flows through us, it gives us the juice we need to feed our physical bodies, our minds, and our emotions, as well as to manage our external environments.

Caroline Myss

What we think, feel, say, and do impacts our body and how it functions. The impact of the mind and our feelings on the body are studied and proven in psychoimmunology.* Medical intuitives, such as popular author Caroline Myss, have seen direct connections between a person's way of thinking and the health of their body. Myss describes some common patterns of this mind/body connection in *Anatomy of the Spirit.*

One way to see this mind/body relationship is through the ancient Hindu energetic understanding of the body and its energy centers, the chakras. The Hindus believed that everywhere, and in everything, there is energy, and it is through particular regions in the body (chakras) that we

---

* *Psychoimmunology or psychoneuroimmunology is the study of the brain's influence on the body, and the body's influence on the brain. Studies have indicated that the psyche/mind plays a role in illnesses such as arthritis, diabetes, and hypertension.*

attract, draw in, and release this energy. They saw each chakra as having a unique location, color, and sound. Disease and physical symptoms in both Hindu and Chinese traditions are understood as blockages, deficiencies, or excesses in the energy flow within the body.

Louise Hays (author, publisher, and healer) has written extensively of her experience with clients highlighting the relationship between their mental patterns and physical symptoms. In *Heal Your Body*, one can look up symptoms and find corresponding emotional/mental patterns as well as suggested alternatives. Through diligent efforts to change her own mindset from a negative to more positive one, Louise healed her traumatic past and cancer.

While my experience with the study of energetics has not centered on the chakras, my healing journey has led me to believe very strongly in the power of the mind/body connection, and the ability to heal the body energetically. As you read in chapters to come (see Chapter 14: *Uprooting My History*), I have experienced a very strong correlation between my "bad thinking" and negative experiences, as well as the contrary.

It is possible to heal through many means. There is no right way to heal. Healing the body is a divine process that can be approached holistically, but not necessarily so. We can heal ourselves by exploring the realms of our minds, bodies, and spirits all at once or focus on one area at a time. Or, we may simply focus our healing in one of these areas. However we choose to heal, whether through the mind, body, emotions, or spirit (or through all at once), we are always healing. And each time we affect healing in one realm, it affects another.

When we understand the chakras and see themes in our lives clearly, we can use this information to better understand our bodies. What so impresses me about this system is how each of the seven major chakras correspond to specific organs, and bodily systems. But what most peaked my interest was their relationship to the endocrine glands (refer to *Appendix 1: Body Basics for CFSers*) and life themes. Because CFS, in my experience, physically impacts the endocrine system far more than any other bodily system, healing the endocrine system is so critical, and the chakra system may provide one path to its healing.

Areas in our life that need balancing may express an imbalance via physical symptoms, through the chakras. When we recognize our symptoms, emotional, or mental imbalances, we can address any of these through various modes of healing. We can, for example, work on changing the energetic pattern through energy work, yoga, breath work, visualization, or bodywork. We can explore our emotions and attempt to change them. Or, we can work on altering our mental patterns. Therapy may offer the means to address our mind and emotions. Whatever approach we choose, we will invariably impact our energy, our overall health, and how we feel.

There are seven main chakras (energy centers) lined up and running through the center of our bodies beginning from the bottom of our torso and moving up to the top of our head. Starting at our genitals, there is the **1) root chakra**. Next, located behind our belly buttons, sits the **2) sacral chakra**. Just below our rib cage we have the **3) solar plexus chakra**. The **4) heart chakra** lights the center of our chest, and the **5) throat chakra** emanates at the base of our throat, where the neck and shoulders meet. Between our eyes radiates the **6) brow chakra**, and at the top of our heads emits our **7) crown/spirit chakra**. Each of these chakras are universally known, yet their names may differ. The chart below, borrowed with permission from Myss (96), *Anatomy of the Spirit*, outlines the organs, issues, and dysfunctions associated with each chakra.

For every chakra, there is an energetic pattern reflected by specific organs and glands located in the body near and around it. Each one also corresponds to various life themes. If

Energy Anatomy	
Chakra	*Organs*
1	*Physical body support* *Base of spine* *Legs, bones* *Feet* *Rectum* *Immune system*
2	*Sexual Organs* *Large Intestine* *Lower vertebrae* *Pelvis* *Appendix* *Bladder* *Hip Area*

Energy Anatomy

Chakra	Organs
3	Abdomen Stomach Upper intestines Liver, gallbladder Kidney, pancreas Adrenal glands Spleen Middle spine
4	Heart and circulatory system Lungs Shoulder and arms Ribs/breast Diaphragm Thymus gland
5	Throat Thyroid Trachea Neck vertabrea Mouth Teeth and gums Esophagus Parathyroid Hypothalamus
6	Brain Nervous system Eyes, ears Nose Pineal gland Pituitary gland
7	Muscular system Skeletal system Skin

Mental, Emotional Issues	**Physical Dysfunctions**

1 Physical family and safety
    and security
Ability to provide for
    life's necessities
Ability to stand up for self
Feeling at home
Social and familial law
    and order
	Chronic lower back pain
	Sciatica
	Varicose veins
	Rectal tumors/cancer
	Depression
	Immune-related disorders

2 Blame and guilt Money and sex Power and control Creativity Ethics and honor in relationships	Chronic lower back pain Sciatica Ob/gyn problems Pelvic, low back pain Sexual potency Urinary Problems

3 Trust
Fear and intimidation
Self-esteem, self-confidence,
    and self-respect
Care of oneself and others
Responsibility for
    making decisions
Sensitivity to criticism
Personal honor
	Arthritis
	Gastric or duodenal ulcers
	Colon/intestinal problems
	Pancreatitis/diabetes
	Indigestion chronic or acute
	Anorexia or bulimia
	Liver dysfunction
	Hepatitis
	Adrenal dysfunction

4 Love and hatred Resentment and bitterness Grief and anger Self-centeredness Loneliness and commitment Forgiveness and compassion Hope and trust	Congestive heart failure Myocardial infarction (heart attack) Mitral valve prolapse Cardiomegaly Asthma/allergy Lung cancer Bronchial pneumonia Upper back, shoulder Breast cancer

	Mental, Emotional Issues	Physical Dysfunctions

5	Choice and strength of will
	Personal expression
	Following one's dream
	Using personal power
	  to create
	Addiction
	Judgment and criticism
	Faith and knowledge
	Capacity to make decisions
		Raspy throat
		Chronic sore throat
		Mouth ulcers
		Gum difficulties
		Temporomandibular
		  joint problems
		Scoliosis
		Laryngitis
		Swollen glands
		Thyroid problems

6	Self-evaluation Truth Intellectual abilities Feelings of adequacy Openness to the ideas of others Ability to learn from experience Emotional intelligence	Brain tumor/hemorrhage/stroke Neurological disturbances Blindness/deafness Full spinal difficulties Learning disabilities Seizures

7	Abiity to trust life
	Values, ethics and courage
	Humanitarianism
	Selflessness
	Ability to see the larger pattern
	Faith and inspiration
	Spirituality and devotion
		Energetic disorders
		Mystical depression
		Chronic exhaustion that is not
		  linked to a physical disorder
		Extreme sensitivities to light,
		  sound, and other
		  environmental factors

we have difficulty in an area of our lives, we may contemplate a life issue/theme and notice if the corresponding organs or glands are affected.

Starting from the bottom of the body, let's look again at each chakra and its associated organs, emotional and mental themes, and associated symptoms.

1) Root Chakra: Immune System

The root chakra is like the root of ourselves, where we

start from the ground up. It encompasses the bottom of our feet up to our lower tummies and includes the base of our spine, legs and feet, rectum, and immune system.

Think of this as the most basic of the chakras representing our most basic needs: our sense of safety, security, home life, and how well we provide our basic needs. When any of these areas are out of balance, they *may* manifest physical symptoms in our spines, feet, legs, and immune systems emerging as low back pain, sciatica, varicose veins, a rectal tumor or cancer, as well as depression or immune-related disorders.

2) Sacral Chakra: Sex Hormones

The **sacral chakra** encompasses the lower trunk: the pelvis, lower abdomen and its organs. It also includes the lower vertebrae, sex organs and hormones, large intestine, appendix, bladder, and hips.

The energetic issues associated with these areas are power and control, blame and guilt, money and sex, and ethics within relationships. When there are imbalances in any of these areas, they *may* manifest as chronic back pain, sciatica, reproductive, or urinary problems.

3) Solar-Plexus Chakra: Adrenals, Pancreas

Imagine this part of your body as the region around your belly button. Making up the **solar-plexus** are the adrenals, pancreas, stomach, abdomen, intestines, liver, kidneys, gallbladder, spleen, and mid-spine.

The energetic nature of this region is expressed through our general sense of self: our self-esteem and respect, honor, confidence, trust, and our ability to care-take. Energetic imbalance in any of these areas may be reflected in problems with any of the organs in this region manifesting as intestinal problems, ulcers, diabetes (and other sugar diseases), adrenal weakness, liver dysfunction, anorexia/bulimia, or arthritis. It is interesting that many illnesses experienced by the CFSer show up here; perhaps issues of self-care in need of attention.

4) Heart Chakra: Thymus, Circulatory System

The **heart chakra**, as its name implies, correlates with the heart and circulatory system, the lungs located around the heart, the ribs that protect it, the thymus and the breasts over the heart.

The life themes reflected by the heart chakra are passionate feelings we often associate with our hearts. The feelings of love and hate, resentment, grief and anger, forgiveness and compassion, and hope and trust are all reflected here.

When any of the above emotions grow stagnant or go unexpressed, they may manifest through physical diseases or symptoms in the heart, lungs, or shoulders. Heart failure or attack, asthma, lung cancer, pneumonia, and breast cancer are all associated with this region.

5) Throat Chakra: Thyroid

Because of the important role our thyroids play in our energy levels, we may be interested in their energetic nature. The thyroid is part of the **throat chakra** encompassing the area around our necks and mouth and including the neck, thyroid and parathyroids, trachea (vocal cords), esophagus (food tube), teeth, mouth, gums, and strangely enough (because it is not located in neck region), the hypothalamus.

The energetic essence of this area is expressed through our dreams, what we want from life, our will, creativity, voice, faith, and decision-making abilities. An imbalance in the throat chakra may manifest through problems in our mouths, throat, or gums. Some maladies associated with this chakra include sore throat, mouth ulcers, gum problems, laryngitis, and thyroid problems.

Personally I have experienced a relationship between a sore throat and either my failing to express myself or allowing myself to cry. In light of my personal struggle surrounding career and meaning/purpose, I find the correlation between the thyroid and the theme "What we want from life" especially intriguing. It is interesting that both sore throat and thyroid problems are common to CFSers, and occur in the same body region. Perhaps themes revolving around the self (our voice, our dreams, and our will) are in need of deeper exploration or attention.

6) Brow Chakra: Pituitary and Pineal Gland

The **brow chakra** encompasses most the organs and glands in the head region. It includes the brain, pituitary and pineal glands, eyes, nose, ears, and entire nervous system.

Energetically, this chakra reflects the feelings we carry about ourselves, in particular: our feelings of adequacy, intelligence, truth, and our openness to other people's ideas.

When we struggle in any of the above areas, our bodies

may reflect this through physical problems in our brains, nervous systems, eyes, and ears. An imbalance, for example, may show up as a brain tumor, stroke, or neurological disturbance. We may experience spinal difficulties, learning disabilities, or loss in sight or hearing.

For CFSers with concentration problems, mind fog, and nervous system challenges (extreme emotions, fear, nervousness, irritability), it may be helpful to contemplate the issues posed by this chakra, namely how we feel about ourselves.

7) Spirit Chakra: Musculoskeletal System, Skin

The **spirit chakra** expresses itself through the very foundations and surface of our bodies: our skeleton, muscles, and skin.

This chakra reflects our spiritual selves, our faith, trust in life, and the service we give. Our values, selflessness, and humanitarianism make up the spirit chakra's themes.

When any of the above spiritual elements are lacking or out of balance, this may be mirrored by energetic disorders, depression, **chronic fatigue** without a physical explanation, or extreme environmental sensitivities.

Beat Fatigue with Yoga, Agombar, Fiona. Hammersmith, London: Thorsons, 2002.

The Healing Energy of Your Hands, Bradford, Michael. Freedom, CA: Crossing Press, 1994.

Heal Your Body, Hay, Louise. Carlsbad, CA: Hay House, Inc., 1988.

Anatomy of a Spirit: The Seven Stages of Power and Healing, Myss, Caroline. New York: Three Rivers Press, 1996.

Gems

However we choose to heal, be it through the mind, body, emotions or spirit (or through all at once), we are always healing. And each time we affect healing in one realm, it affects another.

1) Root Chakra: Immune System – Basic Needs

2) Sacral Chakra: Sex Hormones – Personal Power

3) Solar-Plexus Chakra: Adrenals, Pancreas – Self-Esteem

4) Heart Chaka: Thymus, Circulatory System – Passionate Feelings

5) Throat Chakra: Thyroid – Voice and Dream

6) Brow Chakra: Pituitary/Pineal Glands – Self Assessment

7) Spirit Chakra: Musculosketetal System, Skin – Spiritual Selves

---

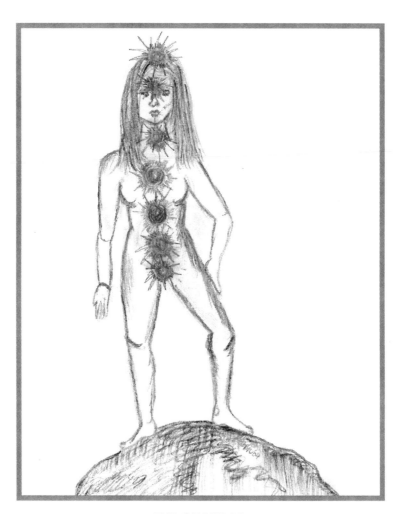

THE CHAKRAS

6
The CFS Tree with Branches Large and Small

Modern western medicine has changed our approach to healing. Body, mind and spirit are treated not as a unity that strives for balance, but as separate entities.

Dr. Edward Taub

Each CFS experience is unique, each with its own story. Yet, at the same time, CFSers share similar physical symptoms and losses, and some may even have underlying issues in common. This chapter focuses on the physiological or bodily symptoms of CFS. (Please refer to *Appendix 1: Body Basics for CFSers* for more on the body and CFS.)

When a patient is diagnosed with CFS, the doctor has first considered the CDC's (Center for Disease Control) definition. If the patient's clinical picture matches this description, then s/he is likely to be diagnosed with the disease. If the clinical symptoms only fit part of this description, then the doctor will likely only diagnose CFS after eliminating all other disease possibilities.

The commonly accepted definition of CFS requires one to have the following symptoms:

1. An unexplained, persistent, or relapsing chronic fatigue lasting six months or longer (not revitalized by rest), and reducing a person's work/obligation load.

2. Have experienced *four or more of the following* symptoms prior to the fatigue's onset and enduring for at least six months:

- significant short-term memory loss
- impaired mental concentration
- sore throat
- muscle pain
- multi-joint pain
- atypical headaches
- unrefreshing sleep
- post-exertion exhaustion (atypical exhaustion lasting more than 24 hours after what was previously a typical amount of exercise)

The above description is only a beginning step for doctors and patients alike to consider whether or not CFS is at work. What you should know, however, is that CFS manifests as so much more than the above named symptoms. In fact, the symptomology of CFS is so wide-ranging that it may appear that the patient has numerous other physical illnesses as well as mental or emotional illness (for more on this, refer to *Chapter 24: Separating Yourself from CFS*). For now, let's consider the most common bodily symptoms of CFS and what they feel like. *[For a very thorough compi-lation of symptoms, see Gellman and Verrillo, (97).]*

To know CFS, to really understand it, you can begin by taking the name apart. The "C" stands for chronic. The most prevalent and pervasive of its symptoms, the fatigue, will last for an extended period: at least six months. Unfortunately, in the case of CFS, *chronic* typically means *years*.

Next, the "F" represents the unrelenting, all-encompassing fatigue. This is not your everyday-variety fatigue that is unpleasant yet doesn't prevent people from going about their business. No, the fatigue in CFS envelops a person—body, mind, and spirit; affecting the body and mind's ability to function. This fatigue is so all-consuming that sufferers feel like they've been run over by a train and no amount of motivation can lift them up. To make matters worse, this fatigue is rarely improved by rest or relaxation. In fact, that is the hallmark of CFS; no matter how tired one is, or how much one sleeps or rests, the fatigue doesn't let up; it's constant, it's chronic. To many CFSers, even simple tasks—from moving muscles, walking, opening the refrigerator, to reading, answering a question, or balancing a checkbook—all become insurmountable.

Finally, the "S." This is the least interesting letter because it simply refers to the fact that this illness is actually a syndrome; in other words, CFS is a recognizable, definable known illness made up of a constellation of symptoms and ailments. CFS is not simply extreme fatigue, but rather it manifests as numerous symptoms and through many other conditions (for example, hypothyroidism, nutritional deficiencies, et cetera).

Though some say that CFS has been around for a century, it was only recently recognized as a valid disease when, in the early 1980's, a "strange illness" (later recognized as CFS or Epstein-Barr) overtook several hundred people in Tahoe, California. Since that time, CFS has gained recognition in the medical field and society in general. However, even today CFS largely remains a mystery. To the doctors who study it, CFS' symptomology is well defined, but its causes and treatments are debated (more on causes at the end of this chapter).

Since CFS remains largely a mystery (in terms of cause and treatment), most people are unfamiliar with what it is. A description of the known, identifiable bodily characteristics of CFS may help friends and family understand the CFSer's plight. For the CFSer who would like friends' and family's support, providing a simple description of the illness may be helpful. Because many sufferers can't quite find the energy or the words to explain their condition, this section may be especially helpful. In fact, it is not uncommon for CFSers to find it difficult, if not impossible, to adequately portray their own experience. Despite the maybe fifty to one hundred symptoms that transform a healthy life to one of chronic fatigue, when asked about one's symptoms, the CFS sufferer's mind may go blank or struggle to access simple words.

I can't tell you how many times I've had the opportunity to explain the illness and wished that I could, only to find that when faced with the moment, I was unable to find the right words.

As I illustrate for you the symptoms and ailments that most CFSers experience, keep two things in mind: *not every person with CFS suffers each of the symptoms below, and some CFSers' symptoms are not included here. [For an elab - orate symptom list, please refer to Gellman and Verrillo (97).]*

Now let's look more closely at the physical side of CFS. The CFS story begins with the obvious: the fatigue. The predominant symptom that changes a CFSer's life is daunting fatigue. However, before the fatigue grows into an everyday phenomenon, a person is typically hit by a powerful **flu-like experience**, a fever alternating with bone-chilling chills, sticky sweats, a painful, raw sore throat, and sensitive lymph nodes—all lasting a few weeks or months.

As time goes by, the flu subsides, and new symptoms replace it. Flu symptoms may come and go throughout the CFS experience or last the entire duration.

While some CFS symptoms are merely inconvenient or unpleasant, others *change* lives. Let us begin our exploration now through some of CFS' "life-disruptors." The first of these is **cognitive trouble**. Before CFS, concentration and the ability to hold a thought and turn it over in your mind was likely never a problem. Now, however, your mind no longer functions as it once did. It's like a cloud has descended upon your brain, preventing thoughts from passing through in their complete form. In addition, your short and long-term memory say goodbye much of the time.

Before CFS, your **memory** failed from time to time, but now you just wish you could remember: where you parked your car, or why you are standing in line at the information desk.

Memory loss makes for embarrassing moments when you can't answer even the simplest questions such as "What can I do for you?" at the bank, post office, or repair shop. When you find yourself in public places bewildered because your mind has drawn a complete blank, and the bank teller is staring you in the face wondering how she can help, then you know that something is not quite right. Your memory has taken a sabbatical.

It's not just your memory that falters; it's also your **ability to concentrate** and **think clearly**. Mental concentration and clarity are compromised. I often experienced compromised mental capacity when I lived in Quebec and would go to the market and have to decide whether to speak in French or English (since it is a bilingual province, with French the dominant language). For me, this shouldn't have been a monumental affair (having previously been an exchange student who lived in France for a year and studied French on and off).

Until the onset of CFS, I could speak French quite well, and years prior, my comprehension had been 100%. During this difficult year, however, I found that CFS radically altered my language skills. Over Christmas, my husband Carl and I visited his great uncle who spoke to us in French. At the time, I concentrated, and desperately tried to comprehend his words, only to find the French jumbled. Three years later, when we visited this uncle again (still having not practiced French), to my sheer amazement, I could easily understand him! The only difference between these two events was a difference in my health and cognitive abilities.

People often refer to the CFS mind as "foggy," an inexplicable veil covers our thoughts, memories, and decisiveness. This **mental cloud** impacts what we can and can't do, making work and study impossible when it involves using our brains for simple transactions and tasks.

Without a brain, a CFSer can lose his/her **sense of self** and ease in the world. If one had been depressed prior to the onset of CFS, now one has more reasons to fall into the pit of despair or *depression*. Often, the mental confusion associated with CFS is accompanied by **emotional disturbances**: *depression, anxiety, irritability, even panic*. It's sometimes hard to know which comes first, depression or CFS. In most cases, CFS precipitates depression, however in some studies, according to *Hoffman, (93)* depression was found to have predated CFS. Anyone who suffers moderate to severe CFS is not only likely to struggle with depression, but has every reason to develop it.

Many of life's most basic functions we all take for granted, are compromised with CFS. The most basic of these is our **sleep**. No matter how important sleep may be for the CFS sufferer, it often eludes us. Either we can't sleep when we need to **(insomnia)**, or we can't seem to ever wake up **(hypersomnia)**, or we simply cannot maintain our sleep because even the slightest of noises jolt us awake **(sleep disturbances)**. Our lack of sleep or sleep disturbances often causes more fatigue and mental and emotional problems. Simply getting many hours of sleep is not enough. We must get deep sleep that goes through four stages. If we consistently interrupt our REM cycle, our bodies will tell us through fatigue, depression, and mental lags. Never underestimate the power of sleep on your physical, mental, and emotional well-being.

Weakness, lethargy, malaise—all epitomize the CFS lifestyle. Nights are disrupted by sleep problems, and days filled with weakness and lethargy. So often this combination leaves CFSers unable to do things they used to do. Even something as basic as getting up, getting dressed, and having breakfast can force a CFSer right back to bed or rest. (Some can't even get out of bed to accomplish these simple tasks.) There just isn't any stamina even for the simplest of tasks.

Just as stamina is compromised, the muscular system screams weakness. CFSers often wake up feeling **achy all-over** or in **pain**. When we wish to walk, run, or lift a box, our arms and legs resist our most simple desire to move, because the muscles are so tired and weak. Many of us suffer from **fibromyalgia** and live out our days in constant, unremitting pain that spikes in trigger points throughout our bodies. Fibromyalgia, while frequently coupled with CFS, is considered its own illness typified by all-over body pain, chronic fatigue, and sleep disturbances (as well as many other symptoms).

Pain can hit anyone, anywhere, but for many CFSers, **pain in the joints** (the knees, ankles, and wrists) can make movement very uncomfortable. I notice my knee pain particularly when walking upstairs. When my knees go weak, they squeak, and crack. I especially notice my knees giving out on cold, wet days—days of grey clouds and darkened moods.

Knee pain and joint pain are not only symptomatic of CFS, but may also indicate **Candida Albicans**, an over-growth of yeast. **Candida** (for short) commonly called **"yeast syndrome,"** is a prevalent illness in today's world of unhealthy refined diets filled with sugar and little fiber. Frequently diagnosed as an infection in the vagina, this imbalance can manifest for men as well as women and can affect the entire body.

Yeast naturally forms inside our bodies and digestive tracts, and when we are healthy, it lives in harmony with hundreds of other microorganisms inside our bodies. However, if we are under stress, or if we consume a diet high in sugar and alcohol, or if we take antibiotics long-term, the yeast can proliferate and ferment, causing inflammation and discomfort. Countless symptoms can be attributed to excess yeast including digestive problems **(bloating and gas), foggy thinking, irritability**, and a slew of uncomfortable, unwanted physical, emotional, and mental symptoms [Refer to Crook, (97), and Martin, (96)].

I highly recommend everyone with CFS explore whether or not yeast is a source of some symptoms. One day, while perusing my Mom's bookshelf, I discovered a book about Candida. Out of curiosity, I filled out a diagnostic questionnaire, and after totaling my numbers, discovered I likely had yeast overgrowth. Most people wouldn't find this good news, but at the time I had been seeking answers to the physical puzzle that enveloped my every cell and to finally see some of the pieces coming together, I was relieved. That day, I began a yeast-free diet, struggling to give up two of my dietary vices, sugar and coffee. I was especially disturbed to discover that I was addicted to sugar, because I was extremely reluctant to give it up. After having finally relinquishing sugar and coffee, and having survived the struggles, I can now enthusiastically exclaim that clearing my body of yeast, coffee, and sugar, were of great benefit to my overall well-being and health.

Candida Albicans, like CFS, is complicated because it, too, has many causes, as well as leads to numerous symptoms, including **food allergies, sensitivities,** and **leaky gut**. Yeast overgrowth in the intestines can cause "leaky gut" syndrome, because it predisposes the intestines to be vulnerable to undigested food particles. This can happen, for example, when we fail to chew properly (or our bodies lack the enzymes to adequately break down our food), and these non-digested food particles find their way down to the inflamed intestine (due to yeast overgrowth). And instead of absorbing the food the way we should, some of the non-digested particles leak out of the intestine, winding up in our blood stream where they travel to different sites in the body. When this occurs, wherever they have landed (whether in the knees or lungs, for example), the immune system reacts to the food particles as the enemy, commanding its army of immune cells to attack. Consequently, various allergic symptoms result, including: **inflammation-like joint pain, abdominal bloating, gas**, and respiratory problems such as **coughing, wheezing,** and **sneezing.**

Candida may also lead to sensitivities in perception (and food allergies). In my first year with chronic fatigue, I was especially confused by the weird "super-like" powers I developed as a result of the physical imbalances from Candida. Later, I recognized these as **hypersensitivity to light, noise, and odors**.

First, my eyes became ultra sensitive. Even the slightest contrast in light and dark caused pain and turned my eyes bloodshot. Every time I went to a movie, for example, I'd come out with painfully tired eyes. Or, if I was in a room with a window, I had to make sure the window was to my side or back so as not to create too extreme of a contrast (between the light from the window and relative room darkness). I became so **photophobic,** that I would impress my then-boyfriend that I could tell if the sun were out even when my eyes were closed! In the morning before opening my eyes, I could always tell if it were sunny or cloudy outside.

My ears and nose were equally sensitive. Loud noises made me jump, and I abhorred being taken by surprise. Odors also became stronger. What once were unpleasant odors, now became nauseating, unbearable odors. For example, while dining in restaurants, I had to stay far from smokers, otherwise their smoke would overpower any enjoyment I might otherwise have. (A good idea for health reasons anyway.)

Loss seems to be the name of the CFS game. If there's something to lose, CFS will find a way to take it from you. Consider the **loss of libido** characteristic of a CFSer. Sex, what's that? Even if you keep your sex drive, you probably won't find the energy to participate as before. It's hard to feel sexy when your energy is shot, your body is weak, and you've gained or lost weight.

During most of my CFS, I've been lucky because I have pretty much remained stable weight-wise; however, recently that changed, too. Just as other symptoms have finally left, weight has gained its way onto my body, and with it whatever sexiness I once felt, now that too is lost. While weight gain makes sense in light of my low-functioning thyroid, that fact does not make my loss any less real.

Weight changes in general likely result from metabolic fluctuations due to a weakened endocrine system. Weight gain may be attributed to a slower-paced life and reduced metabolism or to hypothyroidism, a reduced functioning of the thyroid glands.

Our **endocrine (hormonal) systems**, made up of seven glands, control countless bodily reactions: our metabolism, immune function, sex drive, reproduction, and energy levels. In the CFS patient, endocrine glands are frequently amiss. (For more in-depth information on the endocrine system, read *Appendix 1: Body Basics for CFSers*.) We may suffer **adrenal weakness**, over or under-active thyroids **(hypo/ hyperthyroidism)**, and hormones that are out of whack. Our thyroids determine much of our immunity, energy levels, and metabolism. Our **adrenal glands** respond to stress-levels, either by helping us to cope in difficult situations (when they are healthy), or causing us to panic, when they are unhealthy. The adrenal glands respond negatively to caffeine consumption because the stress causes them to release excess adrenaline. This, in turn, wreaks all kinds of havoc of its own. *[Please refer to Lark, (93)]*

Many CFS patients experience unusually **low blood pressure,** with some exhibiting a unique form called, neurally-mediated hypotension (NMH). Some researchers have discovered that when a CFS body is tipped on a table and then quickly returned to standing, that the heart doesn't pump quickly enough. This causes the blood to remain in the limbs never reaching the brain. The result is **dizziness, inability to think,** and clumsiness.

Not all of us have this type of low blood pressure, yet we may still experience some of these symptoms. I notice that after sitting for a long period, if I get up suddenly, everything twists for a few moments, and I am temporarily blinded for a few seconds—there I am, in the darkness, with a few dots of light piercing through. What is actually transpiring is the blood and oxygen levels in my brain have decreased, temporarily malfunctioning.

Hypoglycemia (low blood sugar disease), is a modern day illness resulting perhaps from unhealthy diets (excessive sugar and refined foods) and the stress we have placed on the adrenal glands do to our fast-paced, stress-filled lives. We usually experience symptoms (resulting form hypoglycemia) after eating a carbohydrate-laden meal, or missing a meal. When the body's glucose levels fall (as in hypoglycemia), the body grows listless, the mind foggy, and in severe cases, **anxiety, panic,** and even **seizures,** can result.

Emotional imbalances, such as inexplicable tears, inability to cope, and irritability, can all be due to sugar imbalance crashes. In fact, a very helpful book, *Nutrition and the Mind, Null (95)* illuminates the important relationship between diet and illness, and explains food-related emotional upsets, including those caused by hypoglycemia.

Also common to the CFSer, are digestive disruptions ranging from **difficulty swallowing, nausea,** to **constipation, diarrhea,** and **gas.** Some of these stem in part from Candida, while others are a result of **food allergies/ sensitivities,** or hormonal and emotional imbalances.

Before CFS, I hardly knew the telltale symptoms of an unhappy intestine. Sometimes I had experienced a little heartburn or gas, but rarely. Unfortunately, CFS led me down the uncomfortable road to **intestinal problems** from A to Z. I'll never forget the time that my intestinal pain and discomfort led to shame and embarrassment.

Carl and I were staying with a friend, and my intestine decided it didn't want to let go of anything. My tummy expanded and grew painful, and Carl, much to my dismay, broadcast to his friend that I was constipated. Having never experienced it before, I was devastated by his indiscretion. It was bad enough that I couldn't get anything to come out of me, and worse when Carl couldn't keep the information between us. After some time, I realized that **constipation** was not a rarity, and I became more comfortable talking about it.

Until recently, I suffered almost daily from indigestion and bloating. I discovered, however, that by straightening out an imbalanced progesterone level and making dietary changes (for example, decreasing caffeine, and supplementing with magnesium and evening primrose oil) helped to eliminate bloating.

No part of the CFS body seems spared from dysfunction. Some of us suffer from **weakened nails, skin conditions, dry hair** and loss. **Hair loss** can be traced to endocrine imbalances in particular, hypothyroidism, and nail and skin conditions could be related to nutritional deficiencies or toxicity.

A final problem for CFSers that I wish to briefly mention here is the vulnerability to additional viruses. Due to a **weakened immune system**, our bodies' ability to fight off viruses is compromised. Consequently, we are more susceptible to colds, flu, and all illness.

CFS truly is a complex illness involving all bodily systems and manifesting through hundreds of symptoms (see *Appendix 1: Body Basics for CFSer*). To gain a comprehensive view of the physical, symptomatic side of CFS, I highly recommend *Gellman and Verrillo, (97)*; or to make sense of the numerous underlying causes and learn ways to heal, refer to *Teitelbaum, (96)*, *Lark, (93)*, or *Murray, (94)*.

CFS Causes

What makes CFS so challenging to its sufferer and doctors alike is the enormity of symptoms and how their causes intertwine. Consider this: many CFS symptoms can be traced to more than one physical condition/source. For example, all CFSers suffer from extreme fatigue, yet the source varies from person to person. Some, for instance, may have hypothyroidism, a major cause of fatigue. While others, may experience insomnia or sleep disturbances, hypoglycemia or candida, food allergies or adrenal weakness, or some, or all of these simultaneously. Every one of these conditions is common to CFSers, and every one can be a source for fatigue.

A helpful way to understand CFS, its many roots (causes), symptoms, and their interconnectedness, is to imagine CFS as a tree (See the illustration: *the CFS Tree*). Alternatively, consider *Teitelbaum's, (96)* view of CFS as a cyclical disease caused by several simultaneous factors (triggers). He links the "feedback cycle" in CFS and fibromyalgia to five sources that trigger fatigue in patients: 1) poor diet, 2) viral infection, 3) trauma, 4) chronic stress, and 5) anxiety/depression.

The cycle begins when a poor diet leads to nutritional deficiencies, and in turn causes loss of absorption. This leads to auto-immune dysfunction and weakened adrenals/thyroid. The adrenal/thyroid weakness then causes fatigue and fibromyalgia, as well as further immune dysfunction. The immune dysfunction, in turn, leads to food and environmental sensitivities that create a susceptibility to infections (especially yeast, parasites, and sinus) which, in turn cause more nutritional deficiencies, cycling once again back to fatigue.

While there are many theories on CFS causes, most doctors recognize the role of viruses, immune dysfunction, environmental toxins, and stress. Some add hormone deficiencies and genetics to the list. In my experience, all of the above seem to play a role (except possibly genetics), but most important of all is the fact that CFS is attributed to many simultaneous causes all of which need to be addressed.

Crook, William G. *The Yeast Connection Handbook*, Jackson, TN: Professional Books, Inc., 1997.

Fischer, Gregg Charles. *Chronic Fatigue Syndrome: A Complete Guide to Symptoms, Treatments, and Solving the Practical Problems,* New York, NY: Warner Books, Inc., 1997.

Gellman, Lauren M. & Verrillo, Erica F. *Chronic Fatigue Syndrome: A Treatment Guide,* New York, NY: Saint Martin's Griffin, 1997.

Hoffman, Ronald L. *Tired All the Time: How to Regain Your Lost Energy,* New York, NY: Pocket Books, 1993.

Martin, Jeanne Marie & Zoltan, Rona, MD. *Complete Candida Yeast Guidebook: Everything You Need to Know About Prevention, Treatment, and Diet,* Rocklin, CA: Prima Publishing, 1996.

Jacob Teitelbaum, MD. *From Fatigued to Fantastic: A Manual for Moving Beyond Chronic Fatigue and Fibromyalgia,* Garden City Park, NY: Avery Publishing Group, 1996.

7
CFS FROM THE INSIDE

True Peace comes from within.

Rosemary Altea

The only way out is through.

Goethe

I write this chapter to those of you who are friends and family members of a CFSer and to you who are seeking a better and deeper understanding of what CFS feels like from the inside. This chapter is also for the CFSer who would benefit from witnessing the inside struggle of another sufferer, thus helping him or her to not feel alone in the challenge. Most CFS sufferers know pain, isolation, confusion, and loss, but few may realize there are others out there who share similar struggles. If knowing my experience helps anyone in dealing with CFS, than my story has served its purpose.

My story is like many, the many dark secrets of lonely, misunderstood chronic fatigue syndrome sufferers. We live everywhere but go unnoticed. We share similar struggles, but are alone. Isolation is inevitable. It's also probably an aspect of every ill person's existence. I don't know. What I do know is CFS; how hard CFS is, and I tell the tale for many—many who are too worn-out, too sick to lift a pen, and too ill to open their eyes and focus their minds. I write for them, I write for you, and I write for me. I write to explain what it feels like *inside* CFS. I write from the nether regions of CFS where illness is all that exists. I write about where I once was, and I write about the worst of CFS, and how it can feel.

When CFS was my life, I was at my worst. (Of course, understand that there are CFS sufferers out there who are worse off than me. My experience, thankfully, is not a worst-case scenario, but it is sufficiently dark to illustrate the hard side of this illness.) When CFS was my life, I was in my first year of marriage and living with my husband, Carl. This was our first year living together full time, and ideally, should have been a wonderful year. In reality, it was the darkest of years.

During this somber period, my life revolved around very little. Each day I slept around twelve hours, often waking in the middle of the night overheated. I'd throw off the covers and tear off any clothing I was wearing and run down the stairs to spit out the mucous clogging my throat. Every morning, no matter how much I had managed to sleep, I would get out of bed (and I know some of you cannot) and very slowly shower and dress. In the shower, there were days when I had to brace myself against the shower wall in order to remain standing. Once dressed, I'd have a nice large breakfast. (Breakfast has always been a very important meal to me.) This part of my day was usually okay because the reality of what I could and could not do had yet to set in.

The rest of my day pretty much involved keeping the house clean, eating, cooking dinner, and trying to figure out my illness. The fact that I was even able to clean and cook is something, because many with CFS cannot. From 7 a.m. until about 7 every night, Carl, my husband, would be far away, at work. In the winter, when he couldn't bike to the train station, I had to get up early to drive him there. This proved especially challenging because of my unpredictable and unrefreshing sleep, but I would get up anyway.

During this year, we lived in what appeared, a paradise. Our small home overlooked "The Lake of Two Mountains" in Vaudreuil, Quebec (just west of Montreal). With few other homes around, situated several miles from two small towns, imagine a secluded, quiet place far from people, desolate, and bitterly cold. To get anywhere driving was required, and for me this task proved monumental. Our van seemed to feel the same way, breaking down as often as I would. So, with a life of going nowhere, except for an occasional errand to the small village of Hudson, I lived out most of my days at home.

During the day, I was always alone—physically as isolated as one can get. (Isolation is an inevitable aspect of illness, but my isolation was also circumstantial due to where we were living.) All I had for company were my two wonderful cats and myself, but mostly, I had myself and mostly, I was not very good company to myself. I was depressed. Here I was, newly married and I hardly ever saw my husband. Each night when I finally did see Carl at the train station, I could barely talk. I was so tired, irritable, and depressed and in my fragile state, I was afraid to even look at Carl. It was as if everything that was hard was somehow his fault. I knew that if I opened my mouth, only pained words would form, so I often chose to keep them at bay. All I really wanted was to eat, watch a video, and then collapse. Our communication was strained, and my one human companion couldn't understand me at all. Not that he had a lot of energy either after working 12-hour days. We both felt cheated and exhausted. I felt it was especially unfair that with what little energy I did have, I used it on house cleaning and food preparation, and Carl felt frustrated by how little I could be there for him after he had spent all day working. All in all, the combination made for two unhappy, tired people, both feeling misunderstood and lost.

Chronic Fatigue Syndrome is an invisible, insidious illness that strips away human vitality. Vitality is essential to a person because it is what makes us feel alive; it is what makes us tick. CFS is invisible because the symptoms are hardly recognizable to outsiders (in many cases, anyway). Despite the ever-growing numbers of CFS cases—now nearing a million; the disease is hidden from the vast majority of us. As a consequence, CFS is very hard to understand, appreciate, or accept for outsiders.

If before CFS you were a painter, now your arms ache too much to lift a brush. If you were an athlete, today you cry because even walking is toilsome. If you were an executive, now you've lost your edge to go, go, go and interact all day with potential clients; now you hardly even want to talk at all. If you were a writer, your ability to think, be inspired, and create have been wiped out. For any of you, you are no longer able to be who you once were. You are no longer able to do the things you once loved. You are no longer able to act in ways you once did. You no longer want the things you used to long for.

CFS robs you of everything you once were. Identities are shattered. Relationships altered. People don't understand. Many of you look the same, showing no outward appearance of illness, and your symptoms elude others. In fact, your symptoms may even elude you.

On a good day, you can forget that you even have an illness, and in all your excitement at having regained lost abilities, you do too much, and then CFS re-ignites, rearing its ugly head and you fall back into bed and realize regrettably what you have done. You suffer days of setback—*relapse*, some call it. Collapse is more like it. Total collapse.

Your whole world collapses when CFS has a hold on you. Every aspect of your being is altered by its powerful (yet elusive to the outside world) presence.

I have never been so alone as I was with CFS. Being alone can be a blessing, but for me, I was deeply lonely, and my loneliness contributed to an ever-growing CFS-induced depression. I lived a non-existent life, one empty, save my daily routine and chores, which I did only because I knew if I didn't do them, they wouldn't get done, and I couldn't bear the idea of living in a mess. It was bad enough that I was a mess! If I couldn't keep myself together, I vowed to at least keep my home together. At least I could maintain some control over my home environment even if I couldn't seem to get a handle on anything else. I felt so out of control. My emotions were unpredictable, my body unreliable, and my mind only worked part-time. Even worse than the physical malaise, were the chronic brain lags. I might open a book, for example, only to realize my inability to read a single paragraph. Or, I might read the words but be unable to process any of their meaning.

When I went out my brain functions would often fail me to the point that I would get lost in the parking lot, unless I had thought enough in advance to map out where I had parked.

When I went to the bank or for an appointment and was faced with a teller or receptionist who asked me what I needed, suddenly it was as if a circuit in my brain had switched off. I would stand speechless, hopelessly embarrassed, waiting for my thoughts and words to be processed. Poor concentration, disorientation, and forgetfulness all had their way with me. Each time I would experience any of these mental dysfunctions, anxiety would usually follow on their tail, and depression not far behind.

No matter where I went, fatigue followed me and with it, a strong desire for retreat. Each time I drove into Montreal (an hour from our home), fatigue would strike so hard that I would have to nap in the back of our van, and I would lay on the floor so as not to be seen. Fatigue made me want to escape, escape from people because I never wanted them to see just how debilitated I had become. Moreover, I did not want them to witness my frustrated cries for fear of further humiliation. On top of that, even the simplest interaction would cause anxiety because I feared going mentally blank, and this made communication impossible. People did not understand, and I was in no position to explain my situation to them.

To illustrate my typical debilitation, let me share a story. One night when I drove into Montreal to meet Carl, all I desired was to be home, in bed—but with both an hour away—I decided to pass the hours away in a theatre while Carl met with his supervisor. Once inside the theatre, when I reached my seat, I collapsed into it. When the movie finally ended, I stumbled off in the direction of the first exit sign I saw. I was supposed to meet Carl at the exit, but had no idea which was the "right" exit, nor did I have the energy to care. My exhaustion was so complete that I was a walking zombie. When I arrived in what appeared to be a lounge, I crumbled to the floor and awaited Carl's rescue. Little did I know, there were several exits and foyers in this theatre, and I had chosen one at the back, not the front, where I had agreed to meet Carl. After much investigation and frustration,

Carl found me. Later, we both laughed.

So much of that year I merely existed with fatigue's grip reducing me to a shell of myself. Even after long nights of slumber, I consistently awoke "unrefreshed" and still longed for sleep. I felt so dead upon waking that I constantly longed for the comfort of sleep.

Fatigue of the constant variety was not my sole complaint. I was hypoglycemic, had mucous clogging my mouth every morning, tongue was coated, and clear, painless bumps dotted the inside of my mouth. Constipation was frequent. Insomnia occurred nightly, and my exhaustion worsened after exercise. Muscle weakness made even the simple tasks of getting dressed and showered an ordeal. Poor concentration and weakened short and long-term memory were daily events. Not surprisingly, I was depressed and to top it all off, had lost my sex drive. For this time, CFS was my life, and I was it. Nothing else mattered. Nothing else existed.

Whenever I could, I desperately tried to read books about CFS and related conditions. I even tried to take classes, but because my ability to function fully for any extended period of time was minimal, this eventually proved impossible since most of the classes offered were far from our home or early in the morning. Since I never knew when or if I would feel okay, I couldn't commit myself to being anywhere for anything. So I didn't. This lack of activity in my life further shattered my already ailing self-esteem. And strangely (in spite of how CFS overtook my life), my family

shared in their doubt my reasons for inactivity, and I sometimes shared their doubt for my non-committal nature.

The consequential isolation created by my illness as
well as the location of our home meant few people saw
me. Except for Carl (who was away at work most of the time),
and my two cats, no one lived with me on a daily basis, no
one was there to actually witness who I had become with
CFS. No one really understood how non-existent I had
become. They just knew that I rarely called anymore, but
maybe did not realize the reason why—I couldn't.

By each evening, when others could be reached by
telephone, I had grown non-communicative. My mind just
could not process in a way that facilitated speech. For me,
a talker by nature, this was a dreaded change.

CFS changed me. It changed me in countless ways.
Before CFS, the first word to pop into my head as a self-
descriptor would have been "energetic." Next, would have
been "passionate," then maybe "athletic." After CFS, I was
none of these. CFS had robbed me not just of my energy,
but the energy that had fueled my passion and athleticism.
All of the sudden, I was a hermit and CFS was the thief who
stole my identity and my life.

GEMS

As a CFSer, you are no longer able to be who you once were. You are no longer able to do the things you once loved. You are no longer able to act in ways you once did. And, you no longer want the things you once longed for.

CFS robs you of everything you once were. Identities are shattered. Relationships altered. People don't understand. Many of you look the same, showing no outward appearance of ill - ness—your symptoms eluding others.

CFS changed me. It changed me in countless ways.

Energy, I Envy

You all seem to have it,
society extols it.
We take it for granted.

This energy you love,
I envy.
This energy
is the essence to
every presence.

Without energy
creativity wanes,
ideas struggle to thrive.
the mind
cannot retrieve meaning,
explanations.
Sometimes the fatigued mind
feels completely shattered,
no longer.

Energy breathes behind all ecstasy
behind the crying child
whose whimpers tell of her yearning.

A no-energy being
can barely feel.
Feelings require so much energy.

When robbed of energy
it's like
the higher beings have robbed me of everything;
all that was and is, me.

I try so many times to
regain my previous life-breath:
sleep more, explore new diets
more caffeine, less caffeine
exercise, peace and rest
low stress
therapy
herbal extracts and teas
traditional doctors;
every conceivable avenue of energy-giving
healing.

But as you can see
nothing feeds me that energy
I so envy.

It seems my lesson is
to learn to live fatigued.

I look around me
and sometimes I buy society's myth;
"do this and you'll be happy."
I try so hard
to keep up with those

all around, those I love,

those with energy.

Then, I pause,

turn

and Sage* greets me

in all her peace,

her essence not energy,

but love.

Sage, my example of what one can be

without energy;

what's meaningful.

Bless you, Sage.

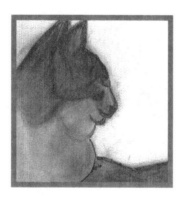

*Sage was my best CFS companion and my very first feline. When I think of her, I smile because she brought me so much joy, and I tear up because I miss her.

8

CALL FOR SOULWORK

Observance of the soul can be deceptively simple. You take back what has been disowned. You work with what is, rather than with what you wish were.

Thomas Moore

So why is it that CFS comes into so many people's lives? Is there some meaning to its presence? If there is, what is that meaning? These are the questions that have plagued us, questions begging to be answered. Questions many of us believe cannot be answered.

I continue to unravel the meaning behind my illness as my journey unfolds. Sometimes I see connections between symptoms and imbalances (fatigue due to hypothyroidism and "raciness" due to yin deficiency, for example) Other times, a way of thinking about an event reveals a pattern repeating itself through physical symptoms. Still, there are other times I decide what purpose a certain symptom has for me; if only to give me the opportunity to be more patient or learn to trust. It's not that behind CFS lies one meaning, but rather that CFS' meaning lies in the journey of the soul. CFS is a *Call For Soulwork*.

Chronic Fatigue Syndrome has entered your life as far more than the illness you experience. CFS has arrived to be your teacher. The message it bears and its purpose in your life are unique to you; you create and define the confines or the vastness of its meaning.

There comes a time in most everyone's life when one begins asking the *big* questions. *Why am I here? What is my purpose? Is there meaning to all of this?* For some, a mid-life crisis will be the catalyst for such questioning. Others have pondered life's meaning and mystery from a young age. Still, others never dare to question, never dare to ponder.

These are critical questions. Our questions about the meaning of life, about the meaning of *our* life, invariably cultivate different answers at different times, changing as we change.

It was CFS that prompted me to deeply consider these questions. CFS stirred my thinking, shattered my identity, and transformed my priorities. CFS catapulted me into soul-searching. No longer could I define myself through what I did, my accomplishments, or where I lived. No longer could I see myself as energetic, athletic, and enthusiastic. No longer was I a people-person who frequently talked on the phone and loved small social interactions. No longer could I afford to believe that I knew what was best for me. In fact, all the seemingly negative changes CFS invited into my life I now know, in hindsight, have been a blessing.

CFS is not about punishment. We are not its victims. We can actually benefit from this illness if we allow CFS to become our teacher. CFS has taught me the most important lesson of all: I am a good person. I don't need to do anything to prove that. CFS continually provides me with opportunities to appreciate myself simply for who I am.

For example, because of CFS I have learned to trust my assessment of my body; I have realized I can heal myself, and I have discovered my passion for being a "health detective" and that I am good at it.

We all have expectations and conditions with which we imprison ourselves. We expect things from ourselves and from others. We have grown up in a work-ethic society where the most prevalent question is: "What do you do?" Is what I do really all that important? When I am on my deathbed reliving my past and readying myself for my passing, will I focus my attention on my life accomplishments? No, I doubt it. I certainly don't believe that is where my mind will go.

What truly matters, and what I will think about, will likely be the love I feel, and the love surrounding me in that moment via my relationships with those dear to me, as well as joyful past experiences. I won't be counting my accomplishments, awards, or the degrees I have earned. What will matter in my dying days is what really matters now: love...love both given and received. What will matter is not what I did with my life, but rather how I interacted with everyone and everything. The CFS teaching here is: my life is about how I live, not what I do.

89

If you have never contemplated the meaning of your life, now may be a good time to do so. If you haven't experienced what *being* is all about—now is your chance. If you have addictions or behaviors you want to change—*now* is your opportunity.

I don't have the answers to your life's questions. I cannot tell you exactly why CFS entered your life, and I doubt there exists a singular reason.

Reasons abound for CFS entering my world. CFS, first and foremost, did not come as my enemy. CFS has something more poignant to offer. It came into my life as a *Call; CFS is my Call For Soulwork.* CFS is my *Call* to look beneath the thick intertwining branches of symptoms, to examine what I believe, what I choose, what I eat, and to know who I truly am. CFS is my *Call* to re-invent and rethink myself anew. CFS is my teacher who challenges me to look beyond the obvious, the unwanted symptoms and question their purpose, meaning, and roots, while simultaneously accepting CFS as a beautiful gift, a teacher, and a *call* to change. *Could CFS have a similar role in your life?*

Could now be your chance to realize never-before discovered parts of yourself? Are you living in ways that you want to change but have been too fearful or too busy to take the beginning steps to address?

CFS is a *call.* It's a *call* to encounter yourself in some new way. Consider CFS a blessing, and it shall be so.

GEMS

CFS has arrived as your teacher. The message it bears, and its purpose in your life are unique to you; you create and define the confines or vast - ness of its meaning.

CFS' meaning lies in the journey of the soul.

CFS is your call to examine your beliefs, choices, diet, and to know who you truly are. CFS is your call to re-invent and re-think yourself anew.

9

EMBRACING ILLNESS

You don't heal from something you are afraid of; you heal toward something you deeply desire.

Dawna Markova

Healing begins when you embrace your illness. Embracing your CFS involves a deep acceptance of your illness, and of yourself in your illness. You may think of acceptance as surrender, giving up the fight to cure an ill. Embracing illness, accepting it fully, means nothing of the kind. You can accept where you are, and still want to be somewhere else.

Embracing your CFS brings peace. When you accept CFS, you are in effect accepting a part of yourself, because you are no longer blaming yourself, shaming yourself, or frustrated with yourself for not being able to do the things you once could. You are no longer embarrassed by your forgetfulness, your inability to focus, your mind-fog—all of your current CFS symptoms. Your symptoms in their physicality are no more than simple facts about what is going on inside you right now. You accept that they are nothing to be ashamed of, nothing to be apologetic for, even when outsiders don't understand. All is okay, because when you embrace your illness fully (and I admit I, too, struggle with acceptance of my symptoms), you no longer need other people to "get it." Sure you would love for them to, but your acceptance is not conditional on their acceptance.

Acceptance frees you; it frees you from the need to make others understand, to prove anything, to explain CFS. All the energy you have expended trying to explain, change, and reframe other people's minds about your illness is better spent on you. *You* are the one who needs energy and attention. It is your body that is clamoring for your attention, asking you to become self-focused for a time.

CFS is your time out. CFS is your illness, and CFS is your gift. Yes, a gift. In fact, when you embrace your CFS completely, you begin to unwrap many gifts your illness bears. One gift may be that for the first time in a long while, if ever, you are giving yourself attention. It may be that had you not gotten ill with CFS and had continued your previous lifestyle you would have ended up with something far worse. It may be that now you have discovered a part of your never-before seen self. It may be that CFS prompted you to make some significant life changes that you otherwise wouldn't have made. The list of possible CFS gifts is virtually endless. Only you can open your eyes and arms to embrace what CFS has to offer.

When you perceive CFS as your friend, rather than your enemy, then your healing really begins. Your healing

of self encourages a physical healing. Without acceptance, your mind tells your body that you are at war. Mental
rejection produces chemical reactions in your physical
body that, instead of healing, result in biochemical warfare.
People leave war in shattered spirits. Souls are lost in war,
bodies are torn apart, and minds are forever altered.

Healing your mind can heal your body, and healing
your body can heal your mind, but healing the soul begins
with healing the mind and body. Soul healing begins when
you embrace your illness and see it for all its possibilities—
a rare gift, indeed. Each person's gifts are uniquely his or
hers, just as each expression of CFS is unique. What causes
CFS and what heals it are also unique to each individual.
For anyone who embraces CFS, CFS comes bearing gifts.
Trust the process. For the only path to wellness is the path
through illness. This path begins when you accept and
embrace CFS' presence.

GEMS

You may think of acceptance as surrender, giving up the fight to cure an ill. Embracing illness, accepting it fully, means nothing of the kind. You can accept where you are, and still want to be somewhere else.

When you accept your CFS, you are in effect accepting a part of yourself, because you are no longer blaming or shaming yourself, or frustrated with yourself for your inability to do what you once could.

CFS is your time out, your illness and your gift. One gift may be that for the first time in a long while you are giving yourself attention.

Healing your mind can heal your body, and healing your body can heal your mind. But healing the soul begins with healing the mind and body.

For anyone who embraces CFS, it comes bearing gifts. Trust the process. For the only path to well - ness is the path through illness.

10
The Gift of Being

It's not how much we do but how much love we put into what we do.

Mother Teresa

We live in a *doing* society. Everywhere people are busy *doing* their lives. Everywhere people begin their social interactions with the all-important question: *"What do you do?"* What does it mean, "What do I do?" Do I do only one thing? Does what I do define who I am?

Having CFS limits the *doing* in life. During CFS, when asked that same old question, "What do you do?" I have often responded with the conversation-stopper truth: "I have Chronic Fatigue Syndrome, and I spend most of my time trying to understand it and learning how to heal myself." Silence usually follows. People frequently don't know what this means, and do they really wish to. A few braves souls, however, venture to ask, "What is CFS?" and to my surprise, I am always caught off-guard by this, and what I had long-imagined would be an incredible opportunity turns out to be an uncomfortable experience. I then falter as I attempt to explain my own daily existence. I can't believe how difficult it is to find the right words to illustrate my experience. I get frustrated. Later, after having said something I usually feel is incomplete, I realize that I wish I had included something like: "CFS is an illness that changes one's focus from *doing* and teaches one to simply *be*, because not only is doing no longer possible, it becomes clear just how meaningful 'being' is."

What does it mean *to be*? It probably doesn't have any appeal to an outsider who sees you just sitting somewhere doing nothing. To them you may appear lazy, boring, or sick—none of which are attractive or desirable qualities. However, if you are the one *being* and you sit, soaking up all that is always around you, you begin to perceive the beauty in everything!

Try it on right now; just *be*. If it's warm enough to go outdoors—do so and sit or lie down in a comfortable place. Feel the sun's warmth on your face, touch the grass beneath your feet, hear the sweet bird songs, watch the dancing antics of the ants. Your world, our world, is beautiful. Have you been too wrapped up in your pain, in the large branches of your CFS, to notice the rest of what is around you?

CFS calls upon you to stop. Stop the frenetic lifestyle demanded by your peers, your bosses, your families, and most of all, yourself. CFS presents you with a whole new way of experiencing your reality—a reality missed by the busy *doers*. This is a reality not to explore, but one to embrace. CFS demands that you stop, feel, look, listen, smell, and taste life in all its wonder.

We are so much more than what we *do*. We are simply who we are. We don't need to *do* anything. In fact, now we are called upon to stop doing things. CFS asks us to embrace our *being*. In so doing, your healing will progress because you will have accepted the essence of CFS, and one of its teachings.

CFS calls you to stop because right now your body is weak and needs a bona fide rest. Go ahead, let yourself be who and what you are now. When you embrace the gift of *being* your awareness eventually deepens beyond the limited scope of your symptoms, and you begin to see the beauty in you and in everything around you. Being who you are is a wondrous thing even amidst CFS.

GEMS

CFS limits one's doing and brings one into being. Through being, you may begin to perceive the beauty in everything.

CFS calls upon you to stop. It presents you with a whole new way of experiencing life. You now must stop, feel, look, listen, smell, and taste life in all its wonder.

11

THE HEALING ART OF BALANCE

Your business is not to "get somewhere"—it is to be here.

Dan Millman

For everything we do in life, there is the fine art of balance. It seems that in all of nature, as in the lives of human beings, the evolution toward balance is first accompanied by excess in a particular area. And, in an effort to correct that excess, we overcompensate and find ourselves in excess of its opposite. This pendulum swing continues until one day we tire of extremes and embrace some aspects of both, mingling them together to create a middle ground: balance.

Balance is something we know we lack by virtue of the fact that CFS has entered our lives. CFS is an extreme. We can no longer do much of anything, and we are now more in a state of *being* than *doing*. *Being* is a beautiful and nurturing place to be, but it suits us best when it is balanced with *doing*.

Before CFS, we likely lived in the opposite extreme, living life as an incredible, accomplished doer. We defined ourselves according to what we did, what we were able to produce and manage. Then, seemingly from nowhere, from deep within the soil of the invisible workings of the energy surrounding us and created by us, we were shaken by CFS. It shattered our *"doing-ness"* forcing us into the opposite extreme. Now, all we can do is *be*—whether or not we wish to. Our lives swung from one polar extreme, *doing*, to its opposite, *being*. This is how it works in nature, and in our individual lives.

All creatures have a waking period in their day in which their minds are alert and bodies are active. However, none of us, (neither fellow humans or animals of any kind), can maintain wakefulness and activity without the opposite down time for the body. We all need sleep and rest.

Somewhere along the line in our progress-oriented, high-tech world, we forgot the importance of these natural cycles. Today, people work and move through their days and nights at a pace contrary to nature's intent. We've forgotten the restful Sunday, and relaxed, low-key vacation. We feel the *need* to climb mountains, even when we proclaim we are on vacation. It is no wonder that so many of us get chronic fatigue!

Fatigue isn't just the plight of unfortunate CFSers; it is also the most prevalent complaint directed to doctors. People are tired and sleeping less and less. According to AAA, the majority of highway accidents today in America are fatigue-induced. *What are our bodies trying to tell us?*

Society has glorified *doing* and has assigned relaxation, peacefulness, and serenity to monks and spiritual seekers, or (judgmentally), lazy people, not for the rest of us. We believe that our importance is defined by our accomplishments and titles. We're not okay just being who we are, without "proving" ourselves. We have taken the work ethic to an extreme, and now we find ourselves stressed and worn-out.

You and I, with our CFS, in a twisted way, are lucky because we get time off from the rat race. We get to just *be*. By *being* we are helping not only our own weary bodies, but the rest of society, too. We are helping demonstrate the opposite of the *do-do* philosophy, and discovering, hidden in the quiet, the reflection, and the pain, there in being dwells something far more than laziness.

When I was a child, I used to spend every day outside running and playing with my golden retriever, Amica. I loved feeling the earth beneath my feet, inhaling the ocean breeze, and absorbing the bright sun. I was the busy, *doing*, little girl in the family who took after my Mom. I had sisters, too, and they, to my bewilderment, spent most of their free time inside their rooms, reading books and magazines, and listening to records. At the time, I just couldn't relate. "Why would you want to read about someone else's adventures, if you could be having your own?" I wondered.

Now I look with entirely new eyes, a different perspective, and I see how our family was balanced, made up of two of us out in the world creating and *doing* life, while the other two stayed indoors, *being* with minds open to imagined worlds created by others.

As I grew into a young woman, I continued to be the

adventurer, the world traveler. Fearless and curious, I traveled to France, Columbia, and Thailand, each time thirsting for the taste of another culture, and sharing adventures with friends. At home, I went to school and worked as a florist. Surrounding myself with flowers, big buckets of water, and lots of people who wanted beautiful bouquets, I thrived under the stress created by personalizing floral arrangements for each customer. Coffee buzzed through my veins, and I felt invincible and on top of the world. Running this way and that, lifting plastic water-filled containers and readjusting sun umbrellas, I was energetic and alive, and I loved it.

My identity depended upon my body's ability to go all day—standing, running, lifting. My sense of self depended heavily upon sun-filled California days, a flower job, and school, and it depended on my *doing* all the time. At the time I was content and I did not realize how much of who I was depended on the external things in my life—my travels, job, as well as my busy routine—my life of *doing*. It only became apparent to me when I found myself too exhausted to go to work, and eventually had to quit school. When CFS knocked on my door, and demanded I stop all the *doing*, it was time for *being*.

Although we all create a sense of ourselves from our external choices, it's important that our sense of self is not dependent upon any of that. Balance is about knowing who you are as part of, and separate from, your family, job, and where you live. Balance is about a life filled with activity and times of calm.

When all those externals in your life are whisked away and you're left facing a stranger in the mirror, you know that your life has jolted out of balance. And now, the CFS that seemingly robbed you of everything is actually what can help you find a new balance between externals (family, job, home) and internals (serenity, reflection, and connection to spirit). CFS can help you balance the *doing* part of life with the *being*. It is in this delicate balance that our soul awakens and our body heals.

GEMS

Balance is something we know we lack by virtue that CFS has entered our lives. CFS is an extreme, about extreme BEING. Being is best when bal - anced by doing.

Society has glorified doing, placing importance upon accomplishments and titles taking the work ethic to an extreme. Now, CFS models the opposite, the significance of being. Balance embodies lives filled with both activity and calm.

12
THE SEASONS OF CFS

In the depths of winter, I finally learned that within me there lay an invincible summer.

Albert Camus

The natural state of our bodies is health. Your body now strives in every way possible to regain balance and to return to health. While health is our natural balanced state, ill health is a statement of imbalance. Everything in life eventually returns to balance, even our CFS-consumed bodies. Your CFS is merely a cycle of ill health, a cycle which eventually circles back to health.

As I write, outside my window a voracious wind thrashes her way through the trees, crashing against windows and thrusting leaves high into the air. Her violent energy disturbs my sleep, challenges the geese, and sweeps the sleeping clouds across the night sky. Though challenging, the wind is a passing friend. She is one aspect of our weather cycle, much like the cold and snow of winter, and the fragrant blossoms of spring.

There are cycles to everything in our lives: our moods,

health, hormones, wealth, economy, and environment. People talk of the stages/cycles of the dying process, of the creative process, of relationships, of human development. Now let's consider the cycles of illness, in particular, yours and mine.

Like the passing wind, the CFSer enters and departs cycles of CFS; it's all part of the natural state of things. The CFSer will probably go in and out of the following phases.

The Denial Stage

A time characterized by the inability to accept CFS.

When CFS first enters your life, you are likely to react with denial, disbelief, or rejection. If so, you have entered the denial cycle, much the same way that people first grieve a death—with an inability to believe or accept the fact of its presence—you do the same with CFS. In not wanting it in your life you dismiss it, pretending it's not there.

Just as the moon cycles in and out of its natural phases, as we begin to heal, we eventually pass through denial into a new phase of acceptance.

The Acceptance Stage

A time to accept there are cycles to CFS.

Knowing there exists cycles to CFS (and to life in general) helps us avoid the tendency toward rigidity. It prevents us from becoming stuck in an unhealthy perception of our illness, and instead we learn fluidity and trust. Knowing there are cycles to the CFS journey reminds us that what we feel now is not how it will always be. The beauty in the cyclic nature of things is: *everything changes.* Life always changes. Remember that in your dark hours. Remember this when you're in pain. Remember it when you are depressed. *Remember that what you are experiencing now is only a passing phase of illness that your CFS tree must weather.*

The Awareness Stage

A time for questioning, seeking, and discovery.

While in, or soon after the acceptance stage, you now enter the awareness stage because now you *acknowledge your CFS.* You see all aspects of your illness, and actively engage with your CFS by trying to understand in-depth what is transpiring and what you can do to heal.

My awareness stage has endured a long time and has been dominated by my desire to understand my illness and do what I can to heal myself. Throughout this stage I've read and studied about CFS and healing.

The awareness stage is also a period for questioning; it is a time of seeking and discovery. It is a time to make sense of the CFS insanity.

My physical inabilities have inspired me to go in new directions and engage in reception, reflection, and learning. This process has empowered me, giving me a new sense of strength when I am unable to find it elsewhere.

In the awareness stage, not only have we come to

accept that we are ill and embrace it for all it is, but we reflect deeply coming to insights that provide meaning to the CFS mystery. These insights further strengthen us, providing us with the courage to face all that CFS brings. As in life, things come and go. Life, like CFS, is filled with cycles. In CFS, these are periodically interrupted by times of un-vitality.

The "Unvitality" Stage

A time to feel hopeless. The incubation period needed for healing.

When symptoms rule and you are caught in feeling low, unmotivated, and demoralized, you have entered a cycle of "unvitality." When immersed in these dark periods, feeling like there is no way out, this is actually a period of rest, a time of incubation, and a slowing down period preparing you for the next stage of healing.

During these more difficult periods, I have felt robbed, grown depressed, become lost, and sunk into a pit of dark despair. Hopelessness becomes my modus operandi as I give into the illusion that my current circumstance is permanent. Many times I think that my situation will never change, but invariably it does. And yours will, too.

When you enter the un-vitality cycle, it's important that you allow yourself to be exactly where you are, even when it feels hopeless. A tree weathers the storm and the long cold winters, knowing that spring is sure to follow. Like all trees, your CFS tree must change with each season. Remember that whatever you are experiencing now will

change like the tree buds that go from nothing to something and from green to gold.

Once you've accepted and embraced your condition,
you can decide to move beyond it and do what you can
to improve your situation. When you have the energy to
grab hold of the darkest cloud and pull it away from your
soul, make the effort. Know, however, that your un-vitality
stage may just be an incubation period or a long-needed
retreat from the world of expectation and excess.

If this is where you find yourself, trust that you must
need this rest. For everything we experience, no matter
how lonely or pointless it may appear, is okay. Everything is
as it was meant to be. All is well. The dark un-vitality
stage prepares your body and soul for another phase of
your journey—the wonderful, light/awakening stage.

The Light/Awakening Stage

*A time to discover your spirit, your connection to others
and the Divine.*

Eventually, darkness always gives way to light. In the
light, you discover your spirit, your connection to others
and the Divine. You may even regain energy and vitality
at this point, discovering purpose and meaning for your
CFS reality.

My light-awakening stage has brought me closer to
Spirit, giving form to an otherwise nebulous spirituality. From
the tunnel of hopelessness where my vitality had van-
quished, I discovered light, meaning, and connection. The

process was a journey, as is all of CFS, with its rocks, pebbles, and boulders along a sometimes treacherous path; but the more I journeyed, the more I learned, and the more I grew, the more I could see my CFS as a blessing.

From the light/awakening stage (where I continue to reside), I tiptoe towards the next phase of my CFS journey, the teaching stage.

The Teaching Stage

A time for sharing discoveries and understanding.

Through this book, I share my discoveries and understanding with you thereby adding more meaning to my experience, and hopefully helping you to discover meaning in yours. As it goes with the teaching stage, you use what you have learned along the CFS path to help others better navigate their own journey. Eventually, the season of teaching leads to the recovery stage, when CFS no longer rules your days and nights and is but a life-changing memory.

The Recovery Stage

A time when CFS is but a memory.

In recovery, CFS is now something of the past, yet the lessons remain. As you return to a healthier life, you fine-tune your life creating one balanced with *being* and *doing*. Now, you are healthy and more evolved because you went through the CFS storm and learned many things along the journey. You are much wiser, healthier, and stronger. But, as in every stage, there are mountains and valleys; here too you may lapse on occasion into old CFS ways of feeling, being, or mindsets. Know that this is okay, and know that the time will come when you take your newly defined self out into the world and reemerge into society in a new way.

Not everyone will enter and depart each of the seasonal cycles of CFS I describe here, but you will move through distinct stages which all come to their eventual end. Cycles and seasons are life's natural order. Seasons offer hope and encouragement because they serve to remind you that one day your CFS will have meaning. And one day you will return to the cycle of health and wellness.

CFS is your body's cycle of imbalance. Its condition asks you to explore yourself, heal what needs to be healed, and care for your body. Your journey has brought you to this CFS tree because something, or perhaps many things, in your life needed attention or reordering. Something was out of balance. Trust the CFS cycles. Balance will return just as the night, in its time, becomes day.

GEMS

The Cycles of CFS

Denial

A time characterized by an inability to accept CFS.

Acceptance

A time to accept that there are cycles to CFS.

Awareness

A time for questioning, seeking, and discovery.

Un-vitality

A time to feel hopeless, yet an incubation period needed for healing.

Awakening

A time to discover your spirit, your connection to others and the Divine.

Teaching

A time for sharing discoveries and understandings.

Recovery

A time when CFS no longer rules, and is a memory.

13
SURVIVING THE CFS LOWS

Be tough in the way a blade of grass is: rooted, willing to lean, and at peace with what is around it.

Natalie Goldberg

In illness, lows are inevitable: low energy, low emotions, and decreased inspiration. Illness is an expression of "lowness," or to put it another way, lack. What begins as a physical lack of energy, transforms into something much bigger—an overall state of deficiency. These are the hard times in one's CFS when CFS rules and symptoms abound. A time when taking "the right action" is hard, and downright unappealing because, after all, one cannot help but think: *will it make a difference anyway?* This is a time when making healthy choices: eating nourishing foods, pursuing healing activities, and thinking healthy thoughts is so important, and yet, so difficult to do.

If you have entered such a low point, I want you to know two things about what's going on. First, this is a temporary state. You will feel better, eventually. Second, it is completely okay that you feel this way. If it weren't, you wouldn't be here. It's that simple. You are here and everything is okay, whether or not you believe that to be the case. At this time, feeling okay and accepting the lows is a challenge, and if you cannot reach acceptance, that is okay, too.

When you are able to accept the lows and are at peace than you have truly embraced the hardest part of your illness. To embrace the low points in your CFS is to help yourself with the natural healing process. Embracing these lows (the uncomfortable symptoms, the sad, angry, or frustrated thoughts, and bad eating habits, for example.) means simply acknowledging where you are, how you are feeling, and what you are doing and saying to yourself. Tell yourself, "It's okay I don't need to change."

Judge not yourself, or your condition; don't fight your feelings, or your current reality. How you are feeling right now is all that really matters. And at the same time, it doesn't really matter so much because it, too, shall pass. Your lows are part of the divine process of your CFS unfolding. This is the eye of the storm. This is the darkest winter before the emergence of the beautiful, bright spring. This is just one of the inevitable cycles of the CFS journey.

Having the lowest of energy; feeling the emptiest we've ever felt; struggling to hold the simplest of thoughts or memories—we can be in any of these states and all the while maintain a sense of complete calm and acceptance. Doing so may not be your first reaction, but after a while, CFS will have given you enough of these moments to help you understand the beauty of surrender. Surrender and embrace. And know that this is simply a passing state; *this is not who you are.*

While deep inside the lows of CFS, it may be hard, if not impossible to explain what is happening because mental and verbal capacities are at their all time low. Now your mind has shut down, your body is frozen, and words are lost somewhere in your ailing mind. This is not the time to try to explain your current condition. You may not even under-stand what is going on. This simply is how CFS expresses itself right now. The time to explain to others about these low states is when you are in a healthier stage of CFS, a more whole state, when communication is less daunting.

I have discovered many times how hard it can be to describe CFS symptoms and the experience of these low states to others. I have tried on several occasions to talk with my loving husband about what is going on inside of me because he just can't see it and therefore does not "get it." Even while we live in the same house, our experiences are often worlds apart.

If you cannot find words to depict your feelings during the rough times, you may want to pick a paragraph or chapter in this book (or from another) that illustrates what you have felt and experienced. During certain stages of CFS, it simply isn't the time to do certain things. When you are at your lowest, it's probably not the best time to try and explain what that feels like. This is one of the supreme ironies of the CFS experience: the feelings and experiences are so real, so overwhelming, and so all consuming, and yet talking about them and understanding them in the moment in which they are occurring is nearly impossible.

At low points, while you may be inclined to seek out others for comfort, this time may be best spent alone. Instead of turning to others during these low times, this is a time to turn *inward*. *Conversations With God: Book One*, Walsch (95) says, "If you do not go within, you go without." This beautiful teaching is one of the many CFS has to offer you.

This is our time to stop everything. This is the time to release our to-do list, our chores, and our judgments. Our bodies need a break. CFS has declared this. That's what CFS is—isn't it?—It is a big break: a break from our past routine, from being superhuman, from attempting to do it all. This is the time to slow down, and perhaps reassess, and re-decide what is important in our lives. Or wait until later to reassess and just be in the moment, doing nothing.

Low times are our time out. They are a manifestation of our body's communication with our mind that we *must slow down and pay attention*. Our bodies are trying to communicate something to us. Maybe we need to change something in our lives. Or, it's possibly a time to change our approach to healing, or simply just surrender to the innate cycle of healing.

Low times are the best times to just *be*. Be present, silent, and do nothing. Be grateful, if you can. Go outside, find a quiet nurturing place, and sit alone and simply rest. Either do nothing and stay with your awareness of everything happening around and within you, or choose to do something mindless, easy, and enjoyable—something creative, perhaps.

When I am low, I frequently sit outside snuggled in my favorite chair and watch the wild creatures and cats do their thing. I am never bored, only entertained by my two furry felines, the squirrels, and birds. I also may take this "alone time" to listen to upbeat or spiritual music. I especially enjoy Enya, Lorena McKennit, Sarah McLaughlin, and Marie Brennan. Soothing harp, passionate vocals, and nature sounds can lighten my dark, low moods or help me to fully experience my feelings just as they are. When my mind is not completely gone, but my body is, I enjoy reading. It can be hard, if not impossible to concentrate, and these times a magazine is a helpful alternative to a novel.

Whatever form of *being* or *doing* you choose at this time, make it one that calls your emotions and spirit to life. Meditation, visualization, yoga, or (in my case) attunement, all serve to bring us in touch with our higher, divine selves. By altering our brain waves and relaxing our bodies, we reach below the surface of our symptoms and make deeper connections with ourselves, and all that is around us.

I just read yesterday (not the first time I've heard this) that spending even a short time in a state of relaxation, (in an activity such as I mentioned above) can replace one's need for sleep. For the CFSer, this could be helpful information, since many of us have difficulty sleeping or getting rejuvenating sleep. Most of us instead experience sleep as non-rejuvenating, remaining exhausted afterwards because we haven't been able to drop into all four cycles of sleep—those necessary for our bodies to process chemical reactions for optimum health. If sleep is a problem for you, as it has been for me, then coming up with relaxing alternatives is vital to your health and healing.

Another way that I like to take care of myself during the lows is through *creativity*. I am a very creative person, but I often let the busyness of life take over such that creativity goes neglected. In the CFS lows, I like to do something creative that I don't have to think about. I let myself create from my intuition and feelings. This is a soul-quenching process that re-invigorates my sense of personal value. Being creative helps me feel good about who I am even when I feel horrendous. For me, creativity may take the form of drawing, painting, photography, or collage. However, it doesn't matter what form the creativity takes because all creative pursuits feed the soul.

So embrace your lows and allow yourself this time to just *be*. Be quiet, surrender, and turn inward. Slow down, pay attention, and do something mindless, but enjoyable. Remember: It's all okay, because this, too, shall pass. Trust the cycle of lows just as you would the passing of a storm.

GEMS

Illness, CFS, is an expression of lack. This is the time to make healthy choices: eat nourishing foods, pursue healing activities, and think healthy thoughts.

At low points, know two things:
First, this is a temporary state.
Second, it is completely okay that you
feel this way.

Instead of turning to others at low times,
turn inward.

Low times are the best times to just be.
Be present, silent, and do nothing.

14
UPROOTING MY HISTORY

At one point I caught a glimpse of myself in the bathroom mirror as I stood up from vomiting and felt such a sudden rush of compassion for the child I saw there… When I lay back down, I had a flash of seeing how the scheme of my life and all the experiences fit together as a congruent whole—a vision that sustains me to this day.

Kat Duff on CFS

Today, I look back through decades past and witness my history; a history wrought with passion and confusion; a history whose path lead, without coincidence, to CFS; a history that now leads to recovery, understanding, and meaning.

I didn't notice boys until I was in the fourth grade. That was okay by me. I was perfectly content to play with my girlfriends, never encountering a boy or thinking about one. Then, one day, one boy interrupted my simple, single-gendered life.

My teacher rounded the class up and we sat in a large circle on the floor, each introducing ourselves by name and sharing a little about ourselves. I remember now, 23 years later, Greg's declaration, "I am Greg and I am the greatest!" I recall feeling a mixture of repulsion and awe at his blatant confidence.

Greg and I shared first and last initials, providing friends with perfect tools to tease. "Greg plus Gretchen," they chanted. I wanted to disappear. When it came to Greg, disappearing was my most desired wish. When we'd line up in alphabetical order and wait for gym class to begin, Greg entertained himself by whispering embarrassing, sexual comments in my ear. I cannot recall his exact words from that time, but I imagine them to have gone something like, "I'd like to see under your panties." Mortified, I would stand in silent embarrassment, shifting from foot to foot. What did he want?

As much as I wanted to hide, later, when physically distant from Greg, I found myself puzzled by simultaneous feelings of aversion and intrigue; I was developing a crush. These school experiences marked the beginning of what I would later understand as male/female games. They looked a lot like cat and mouse with the girl playing the "pursued" and the boy, "pursuer."

As I entered adolescence, my body developed quickly, but my sexuality evolved more slowly, especially for a girl in Mendocino, the small, coastal town where I grew up, (where sex, drugs, and rock n' roll were the rule for the majority of teens). Throughout grammar, middle, and high school, I remained largely disinterested in boys. Most boys seemed equally disinterested in me; occasionally, however sexual comments were thrown my way by older boys. These, it seemed, were always directed at my body parts, not me. "What a piece. I'd like to get some of that..." they'd announce. Beneath my embarrassment, I boiled. I hated being objectified, but felt helpless in the face of sexual innuendo.

As I entered my twenties, my reactions to males changed, and my sexual drive kicked in. What was once embarrassing suddenly took on the flavor of excitement. As if a shot had been fired to begin a race, I began dating any man that took interest in me. And there were many.

Like so many women, I wanted the fairy-tale; I wanted Prince Charming to sweep me off my feet and love me. But having never established friendships with men, and having had few male role models in my life, I knew nothing about love or how to be in love. I convinced myself I was satisfied with my fast-paced sexual relationships. For a time, I was (or so I thought). But as my dates developed into relationships with men more interested in sex than feelings, an emptiness grew inside me. I craved companionship and emotional intimacy. Instead, I experienced brief periods punctuated by excitement, mystery, and sexuality. After these fun-filled weekends, I was ultimately left feeling lonely during the week. Even when I demanded more from my dates, I discovered the same painful truth time and time again—none of the men I dated wanted to give up their freedom. I was a play-thing, someone to use at their convenience. I was the server, the chased mouse, and the epitome of the oppressed. I had become a woman who put a man's desire first, and I felt lonely and used.

After three relationships with men who didn't give a shit about me, I was about ready to call it quits. When I found myself standing outside a boyfriend's apartment, yelling obscenities at his door, begging him to let me in so that we could talk about why he wouldn't return my calls or see me, I realized then and there just how low I'd sunk. When his door slammed in my face, I felt shame well up inside me. It was time to swear off men, at least until I had enough sense to not let one treat me like dirt. I was fed up with uncaring men; a male "fast" was in order.

Thoughts, words, and actions are invisible forms of energy that shape the world we see and the world we per - ceive. Our most constant and pervasive thoughts, words, and actions attract similar experiences to us.

In 1991, I moved from Berkeley to Santa Rosa, CA. After experimenting with art, photography, and psychology classes at Sonoma State University, I enthusiastically enrolled as a psychology major. I devoured theories, applying them to my life. I read and wrote about what interested me: people and their personalities, ways of thinking, and behaviors. The classes I chose in many ways mirrored my life and my unre-solved issues. In class and out, I grappled with my role as a woman and the expression of my sexuality; things quickly came to a head.

On one memorable warm afternoon, the outdoors beckoned me to take a walk. Outside I went, walking from my neighborhood on the west side of the tracks to Railroad square, a refurbished train station and quaint shopping area. When I reached a busy underpass that divided new town from old, cars sped by. I walked briskly inside the shadowy thoroughfare. Once a few feet into the underpass, I noticed the sound of footsteps several feet behind me. The steps, like mine, sounded unusually fast. Unsure what to think, I maintained my rapid pace, as did the person behind me. With every step I planted, one just like it reverberated from behind. Frightened and confused, I quickly stole a glance at the person behind me. He was tall and thin with wavy, dark hair. My breath grew shallow as my heart began to race. Anonymous cars raced by oblivious to the game of cat and mouse that had begun. I tried not to think about much because when I did my thoughts frightened me. To test my theory that the man on my tail was following me, I slowed down as we neared a desolate street beyond the pass. My throat tightened in anticipation. When I slowed, the behind man slowed. One street, then two, I alternated between walking briskly then slowing to a snail's pace. Finally, I picked up my pace again, hoping to shake my follower. When that failed, I slowed to a near stop to let the man pass. When that proved ineffective, I decided to cross the street. Again, he followed. No matter what I did, I could not shake him. My fear grew.

When we finally arrived at Railroad Square, a quaint area filled with boutiques, restaurants, and a café, I thought, *At last I can get away!* I ducked into El Mano

Boutique thinking this would be the end of our game. Only seconds later, the man reappeared. My fear now turned to disbelief, shock, and I debated what strategies to use next. I considered hiding in the dressing room, but instead opted for a quick escape. I darted from the store to an inn across the street. Feeling more like an escaped convict than a victim of a chase, I whispered to the receptionist what was going on. She called for a cab and compassionately showed me into an adjoining room where I could wait. I peered through a crack in the ruby-red curtains and caught sight of my pursuer across the street entering my favorite café. The game had finally ended...or at least this one had.

For the next two turbulent years, I would call a yellow cottage on Iowa Street home. It was situated on the west side of the tracks, in what I later learned was one of the poorer, run-down areas in town. As much as I loved my home, I hated that it was surrounded (on both sides and in the back) by other small rentals. Two couples lived in two of the homes sandwiching mine. Behind my cottage was a tiny studio that housed a single man, Don. While Don became my friend, the other neighbors seemed the sort of characters likely to end up on *Unsolved Mysteries*. In the middle of the night, I was frequently jolted awake by angry screams and loud thuds. Whenever this happened, I huddled beneath the comfort of my blanket, pulled my cat Sage close to me, and grabbed my flashlight to record words barely audible. Alone and scared, I scrawled these journal entries: *My neighbors woke me up again. They are definitely frightening. I heard Tracy scream, "Get away from me; get the hell away from me!" and "I hate you, you fucker!"* A later entry reads: *This time it's not Tracy and her man in a conflict, it's the other neighbors! This is real! I hear glass shattering. Sam comes over and tells us (my neighbor Don and I) that he's sorry to bother us, but his fiancée is berserk. He rambles on and finally concludes that he loves her, but she has threatened to kill him.*

In the daytime while studying at SSU, I read books about sexual assault and incest, pouring through articles about men harassing women—researching connections between the socialization of men and violence against women. I studied psychologists and their theories, including Jung's concept of synchronicity. The more I read and thought about violence, the more I seemed to experience it (inside and outside my home). Synchronicity?*

As my neighbors raged on at night, by day I was the object of catcalls. Whether I sported a short, sexy dress or grey sloppy sweat pants, it didn't seem to make a difference. Walking past a group of Mexican men, hisses and sexual comments shot at me. According to my gender studies text, the words and hisses leaving the men's lips burned with power. "Men don't simply whistle or catcall just for the hell

* *"Synchronicity," coined by psychoanalyst Carl Jung, refers to any meaningful (acausal) coincidence. It may be a meaningful coincidence between two external events, or between an internal (psychological/ mental) experience and an external event.*

of it; they do it because it makes them feel powerful," the text declared.

A year into my studies at SSU, I decided to take the trip my sister and I had always dreamed about. Only I would take it alone. I flew to Europe equipped with a 50-pound backpack and an enthusiastic wanderlust. At 24, I felt as though I had, after several years living alone, conquered doing life alone—all that remained was the experience of independent travel. After having spent an adventurous month with youth hostel crowds of 20-year-olds exploring historic downtowns and ancient cathedrals, hiking pictur-esque hills and mountains, and visiting London, Edinburgh, The Lake District, Venice, and the Alps, suddenly my savory trip took a dive.

It was late when I reached Grenoble and I was tired and ready to crash at the hostel. Outside, rain pounded. A bus dropped a few other backpackers and myself off at the youth hostel on the outskirts of town. Inside my room, bare mattresses waited to be filled with warm bodies. The outside rain dripped through a ceiling crack drop after drop like a leaky faucet. Out of nowhere, a thin, Middle-Eastern man appeared and sat down on a mattress next to mine. As we struck up a conversation in French, I was too tired to realize the fact that he was in a room designated for women. Later, downstairs, he asked me if I would join him for a trip to town for dinner. I accepted.

It was eight p.m. and the rain had finally stopped, but the sky had blackened. I felt my hunger, but had no food.

We grabbed the next bus to town, where I followed the man. I was surprised when I found desolate streets and darkened storefront windows.

What happened next is forever embedded in the cells of my jaw. My companion invited me up to his apartment and I wondered why a backpacker would have an apartment. The inconsistency, however, was too cumbersome to unravel in a language I hadn't spoken in years, and I was too tired to worry about it. I left this thought behind as I followed him up to his apartment on the premise that we were just dropping off his guitar. But once inside, feeling proud that I had recovered my buried French, I conversed casually with him, as he pulled cans from a cabinet and placed a pot on the stove. Soon, I joined him for bland pasta, and after dinner, our friendly conversation ended, and the man I had known for only a few hours turned against me.

Suddenly out of nowhere the man lunged at my body, grabbing at my limbs and torso with his hands. In shock, I tried gathering my belongings to leave, but as he kissed my shoulder he worked to keep me seated. Fighting him, I wrenched myself from his grasp. When he persisted, I grew angry; and my anger ignited a fury in him. To prevent me from leaving, he wrapped his hands around me with an impenetrable grip, covering my mouth. His fingers dug into my jaw. In this suffocating position, he dragged me into the adjacent room.

To this day, I can still feel his steel fingers pressed into my jaw. Luckily, I was a close match for his small frame and strength. Our struggle lasted only minutes, although it felt more like hours. Throughout the struggle, I screamed for help, swearing any French profanity I could dredge up. My attacker reacted with, "Je ne veux faire du mal," meaning, "I don't want to hurt you." After one hell of a fight, my screams and resistance grew too much for my attacker and he let-up. I fled.

I had endured yet another violent encounter, adding evidence to my conviction that men at odds with women knew only to dominate and control them.

As you believe you will experience.

Neale Donald Walsch

It was becoming more and more apparent that as my thoughts grew in their anger towards men, angry men kept finding me. The more danger I faced head-on, the more I felt in danger. It didn't seem to matter that all I wanted was freedom from anger, violence, and fear. Instead, fear enveloped me, seemingly following me everywhere.

Fast-forward two years. After a joyous Christmas break in Montreal with my then boyfriend Carl (whom I had met that fateful European trip), I flew back to California to return to school. I arrived on Addison Street in Berkeley and parked outside my sister Mena's home. Life was good, I felt. I loved Carl and was looking forward to a return to psychology and photography at SSU. I rounded my Celica into a parking space and lifted my luggage from the trunk. I began to make my way across the few yards to my sister's home when I heard a strange ranting. I could barely make out the figure, but knew someone was rapidly approaching me.

Out from the darkness, a thin and enraged man with one arm raised skyward charged toward me. I didn't know what to make of what was happening. In one moment everything that had seemed so ordinary and perfect was quickly transformed into the surreal. A rubber mask, reminiscent of Frankenstein with scars and sharp features, covered the man's face. He carried what appeared to be a gun. In seconds, he was upon me, grabbing and pulling me from the middle of the street. Shocked and terrorized, I hardly moved except to resist his pulls. I was afraid to fight because the man was enraged, perhaps psychotic; and I couldn't help but feel that he might do something horrific and unfathomable. My hand that held my suitcase handle now went limp, and the suitcase fell to its side. There in the middle of the black street, we struggled. The man wrenched me in the direction of my sister's home, and I pulled equally hard in the opposite direction (I was afraid of him pulling me into the bushes and out-of-sight). As we fought, I screamed, and shrieked as if my life depended on it. "Help, Mena! Help, Clint!"

But the street was deserted except for my attacker and me. I kept screaming and tried not to think. I was too afraid to imagine what was possible, but one thought permeated my mind, repeating itself over and over like a mantra, "It's not real; it's not real; it's not real." These words reverberated in my mind again and again as if to reassure myself that everything would be all right. In reality, I felt I was dangling over a precipice and the mad man had me by the hand, the master of my fate. As we fought on, a part of me felt the urge to rage and fling my fists against my attacker, but I couldn't let myself fight hard, because despite my mantra, I believed his gun to be real. Somehow I knew from the moment I saw its shadow that it was real. Yet conversely, at the same time, I had to convince myself it wasn't.

During the attack I had no idea what my attacker wanted. I only finally realized he was tugging on my purse, when the force of our pulls snapped it's strap. It was only then that I realized this was the strangest of muggings. As I continued to scream, nobody came; Mena and Clint stood just feet away inside their home, but they never came. Now, angrier than when he first charged at me, the attacker struck me on the forehead with the gun handle. Perhaps my screams and resistance had exasperated him. The attack was finally over.

Despite my terror during the attack, what followed in many ways felt worse. My sister and brother-in-law had been expecting me. Kay, my other sister, had just called them to let them know I was driving over. While the attack was in full force, Clint stood, watching at the window what he believed was a petty fight between two women he didn't know. When Mena finally opened the door to my blood-streaked face and hysterics, she realized that I was one of "those women." Inside, I collapsed from my hysterics and crumpled to the floor where Mena sat a few feet away emotionally and physically paralyzed.

Internally, I reverted to being a little girl, reaching my arms out toward Mena in a silent plea. All I wanted was a hug, some words of reassurance. But neither Mena or Clint was capable of tending to my needs. They did what they could, calling 911 and reporting the incident, and I did everything else.

I wiped the blood from my face with the wet washcloth Mena handed me. Afraid that I was severely injured, I asked Mena if my cut looked serious. She must have said, "Not really," because I gathered the courage to take a look in the mirror. At the time, my head injury was the least of my worries. Somehow I managed to call credit companies to report my cards stolen; then I described the attack to the police from behind the window of an officer's car peering out the car window at a suspect that had been arrested soon after my attack, and was examined and questioned by paramedics. After all of this (now some time past midnight), Clint drove me to the hospital. From the moment the attack ensued to the many hours that followed, I remained terrorized. It was as if a switch inside my body had been tripped, and nothing could turn it off.

On the way to the ER, Clint said, "You're lucky you weren't killed." The combination of those cruel words coupled with his lack of action during and after the attack, built up a wall of mistrust that to lingers to this day.

One after another, dangerous male strangers haunted me with their violence. Theories I had read, and papers I had written about violence perpetrated by men against women erupted from words on pages, into my life. Internally, I was in turmoil.

Immediately following my mugging of January 21, 1994, I began acting like a Vietnam vet. Inside my house, I hid from the world, tacking up blankets over my windows to keep outsiders from seeing inside—from seeing me (even though I loved natural light). Whenever an unfamiliar noise broke the silence of home, I would scurry into a corner, stop breathing, and crouch in terror—hiding from my imaginary assailant. Every time I walked from my home in broad daylight to downtown Santa Rosa, my heart pounded and my breath grew shallow each time a man passed by. From that point on, I never felt safe anywhere, neither inside my home, or outside of it. But my fear was most pronounced in Berkeley, where my family lived and where I had been mugged.

Nobody seemed to understand what was transpiring, but most of all, not my family. When my Dad first heard about the mugging, he responded, "Gretch, why didn't you just give the man your purse?" Later, when I really wanted to see my sister, Kay, but was too terrified to drive to Berkeley, I called her and suggested we meet somewhere halfway. As if I had asked the world of Kay, she erupted like a volcano and responded with something like, "Gretch, just get over it!"

Aphrodite Matasakis, *author of I Can't Get Over It: A Handbook for Trauma Sufferers, explains how secondary wounding occurs when family members fail to support trauma victims. Unsupportive or negative reactions of family members following the event, exacerbate the victim's feelings of abandonment which were initiated by the trauma.*

A year following the mugging, my life was inundated by Post Traumatic Stress Disorder (PTSD*). Whenever Carl called me from Montreal, he frequently endured long periods of silence as I froze into a flashback reaction. Fear would freeze me—my eyes would dilate, heart race, and my breath became constricted. Mostly I grew silent, watchful, motionless.

After a couple of weeks following my attack, I sat in art class and listened to the teacher describe our first assignment—mask making. I instantaneously knew I couldn't do it. With tear-filled eyes, I told my teacher about the mugging incident and asked if I could substitute mask making with a different project. She made no concession. Luckily for me, somehow Carl seemed to have the answers to my continued feelings of abandonment and misunderstandings; he tallied my school credits and informed me,

---

* *PTSD is a common disorder experienced by people who undergo (or witness) unexpected life-threatening events such as combat, natural disaster, accidents, or violence. Sufferers frequently relive the trauma via nightmares, flashbacks, and may suffer symptoms such as: difficulty sleeping, anxiety, hyper-arousal, feeling detached or dissociating, hyper-vigilance, memory problems, and depression. (For more information go to www.ncpt.org)*

"You can graduate this semester if you give up your art minor." I felt relieved, elated even.

Soon thereafter, I found out about Antioch New England Graduate School, situated in the Northeast, close to Carl's home. When I was accepted into their counseling psychology program, Carl flew to California, so he, my two cats and I, could drive across country to Burlington, Vermont.

Believing that I had left PTSD behind, I was excited about getting on with my life in pursuit of a Master's degree; I was on the way to becoming a therapist! The first half of my year at Antioch went well, academically speaking. Yet, my body had begun to send signals of an underlying disturbance that I could hardly ignore.

By the time the second semester rolled around, I was sleeping 12 hours each night and would wake up groggy to the sour taste of phlegm choking me. At my internship, my eyes strained to stay open, while words blurred from text pages into nothingness. Only caffeine and a brisk noon walk kept me going both at Antioch and the internship. The fatigue grew so strong that I began to question if something was physically wrong with me. Later, I discovered that something indeed was wrong, terribly wrong. That "something" was CFS.

The roots of the CFS tree run deep beneath the rich soil of memory. We, with our most powerful thoughts, words, and actions, nourish CFS. Only when enough of the roots of the CFS tree are no longer nourished, will the foundation on which it relies, decay. Without its roots, the CFS tree cannot survive.

When CFS found its way into my life, I was the frightened little girl all over again. I just wanted big arms to embrace me and take me away from the Frankensteins of the world. But nobody, not even my best friend and future husband, Carl, could save me from CFS. I would have to learn to save myself.

GEMS

As my thoughts grew in their anger towards men, angry men kept finding me. One after another, dangerous male strangers haunted me with their violence. Theories I had read, and papers I had written about violence perpetrated by men against women erupted from words on a page into my life.

We, with our most powerful thoughts, words, and actions, nourish CFS.

15
STANDING ALONE:
THE INEVITABLE ISOLATION

There's only one of us in the room.

Neale Donald Walsch

Before CFS, I lived alone and went to school and returned home from school alone; being alone was a way of life. Much of the time, I felt like I was choosing to be alone and was okay with it, but at other times, I fell into despair: the pit of separation, isolation, and depression. I felt far away from my family despite their physical proximity, and I felt far from the experience of community. In every way, I was alone.

We live in a lonely new millennium with people farther and farther apart from one another due to lifestyle choices and perceptions of the world. No longer do we look to family as a community of support and care. Many of us have replaced our family connection with our partners, our own families, peer groups, or the TV, computer, or books.

We can avoid people-encounters altogether if we choose by: ordering in, cooking at home, having groceries delivered, using drive-throughs, purchasing online, remaining in our cars at the bank, and staying in the comforts, confines, and safety of our homes. It is sad that we have in many ways used the conveniences of technology to promote isolation and separation. The more we stay at home taking in our view of the world through the eyes of television; the more we breed the separation that comes from keeping ourselves locked away; and the more apt we are to perceive our world as scary because that is how the media portrays it.

Some of us who remain alone, watching the news or listening to the radio, wishing perhaps we were out, begin to believe that it is scary "out there." As we spend more time engaged with machines, alone in our individualized universes called home, the more separate we feel.

We are more isolated in our modern technological world than we were 100 years ago when we met our neighbors in the local bakery. Now, if we want, we can go long periods without ever encountering our neighbors, or even our friends. Instead, we've built our busy lives around people we don't necessarily like. At work, we may even feel unrecognized or inadequately rewarded. And arriving at home, tired from a work-week lacking passion and connection, we settle into a comfy couch with our favorite drink, and watch a video to escape a life of separation and loneliness.

Our sense of isolation is more perception, however, than reality. Isolation is the unwanted feeling of intense loneliness and alienation. This feeling is often accompanied by the belief that you cannot change your reality of separation. The belief, however, is simply that: a belief, (not necessarily the truth based on the circumstances of life). Our beliefs, though very real to us, are not necessarily reality. When founded upon past experiences, which are no longer much more than memories, the isolation we feel is, in fact an outgrowth of our mindset rather than reality.

Both separation and connection are available to us and are dictated by the choices we make through our actions and the perceptions we hold. We all have the opportunity to be a part of our world, because *we all are a part of it.* The separation we feel exists in what we believe to be reality, but the universe with all of its beauty and magnificent creatures, are part of the same interconnected entity. CFS, by requiring us to slow down and simply *be,* provides us the time and space to ponder and experience our connections to the great web of life, and to recognize all its splendor.

Isolation, perceived or real, can also result in part due to our physical circumstances. In fact, isolation is nearly inevitable at some point in the CFS journey. Because the medical field remains baffled by CFS, many physicians continue to regard the CFS patient as an unwanted challenge or threat. Some may even assess the chronic fatigue sufferer as having mental problems and refer him or her to a psychiatrist. Yet, despite the catalytic changes our lives undergo, the CFS mystery remains even more elusive to friends and family. They are confused by this unpredictable, invisible illness that silently robs us providing us little physical, tangible evidence of disease that they might be able to understand.

The dark mixture of CFS symptoms creates a nutritious soil for being and feeling alone because others don't "see" our maladies or comprehend the great impact that our symptoms have on our everyday existence. We CFSers may struggle daily with countless symptoms, while those closest to us fail to understand what we're going through because they are not struggling in the same dark soils beneath the CFS tree. The consequence is: separation from society, from community, and from our friends and families.

Though our symptoms do affect how we relate in relationship to others, and thus impacts our friends and families, only we feel the pain, fight the fatigue, are clouded by the mental fog, and suffer the intestinal upsets. Outsiders see that we've had to change our lifestyle; they see that we may not be lively or mentally present, however they don't experience the actual physical aspects of our disease. They simply cannot relate. No matter how much you try to explain, friends and family remain on the reflective side of a one-way mirror—never having experienced the utter disappearance of their vitality; their understanding of our overwhelming fatigue extends only as far as their ordinary fatigue experiences. Consequently, the people in your life can't help but minimize your reality, and they may just want you to "get over it."

Often people don't want to truly understand our debilitation because it means that they too would know what it feels like (and they don't want to feel debilitated). Consequently, by not knowing and not understanding, many lack compassion towards our CFS realities—compassion much needed and deserved.

While others pull away from us due to a lack of understanding or compassion, we also pull away for similar reasons. When family and friends lack compassion, or worse yet, judge us for not being who we once were or who they wish us to be; we distance ourselves. We turn away and turn inward. Feeling rejected, we reject in return. Over time, we separate ourselves emotionally and physically from others— isolating ourselves, we stand alone.

There are many more reasons we may remove ourselves from the company we used to keep. The very nature of CFS weakens our bodies until we become able to do less and less in our lives. We do less for ourselves and less within our relationships. We may leave a job or decrease our working hours, only to come home and crash. We can no longer do what we want to do for ourselves or for our loved ones. At times, we barely function. We simply exist. While in this limited state, we can't understand the complexity of our illness nor can we communicate this to our friends, families, or partners.

In fact, from our weakened state we are more likely to react to others in anger, frustration, or sadness because our bodies are so over-stressed, our nerves are so fried, that everything tends to feel like an emergency. Or, we are just so exhausted, so depleted, and our bodily systems so over-worked, that we grow numb and unresponsive. Either way, we are no longer fun or easy to be around. And while others may not enjoy us as much, we don't enjoy them as much either in this fragile state.

Many relationships are unable to survive CFS. In fact, it is amazing that any relationships do. Thankfully, some survive and are even strengthened by the experience. But for the most part, we retreat and others retreat from us; we stand very much alone in our CFS.

If your family, like mine, lives far away and visits are infrequent and short, CFS can increase the amount of sepa-ration. Living far from one another decreases each person's understanding of the other's daily reality and choices.

I have realized that I am increasingly less comfortable visiting when people expect things from me. My family knows I've changed, but they don't understand it. Frankly, I don't think they want to. At the beginning of any unpleasant circumstance, my family's motto seems to be: *Get over it*. In response, "Nobody understands," became my CFS mantra, and isolation my way of life.

One danger of isolation is that bitterness and hope-lessness can take root in our lives. The remedy is a feeling of connection and hope. Hope extends from the belief that things will get better. Without hope, depression sets in. In order for us to emerge from or avoid depression, we need to feel a *part* of something. We need meaning in our lives; meaning that we ourselves create will likely be different from our former sense of purpose. To create meaning and feel a connection, we need to do something that feels important and enriching. Creation empowers us, and gives us a sense of purpose. Connecting with others or making meaning, can be a huge challenge from a bedroom when we are bedridden or housebound, but it is possible.

Ironically, the technology that tends to feed our isolation can also provide connection in times when we can't help but be isolated. You may want to use the phone more and talk with a supportive friend, or log on to the Internet and chat with others who share a personal interest. If even these activities exceed your current capabilities, you may want to listen to dynamic talk radio, inspiring books on tape (which you can get from a library, if cost is a factor), or watch your favorite TV shows.

Doing anything that helps lift your spirit and inspires you to believe in yourself and your importance in this world, that affirms your connection to the all that is—is time well-spent. Or, you can do nothing and find connection this meditative way. Just *be*; be the CFS tree in the outdoor world of beauty and freedom. Go out in your yard, to a park, or to a favorite nature spot and spend time amongst the creatures and green things of the earth. When connecting to other people feels too difficult or too demanding, animals and nature offer a wonderful alternative to total isolation. Most animals are quiet and peaceful and they live in the present. They don't regret their pasts or worry about their futures; they just are, now. Your CFS requires that you, too, align yourself with animal-nature. It is our nature, too.

Time outside amid the backyard birds, buzzing bees, roaming ants, and frisky squirrels is an easy place to feel a part of it all; it is an easy place to return to peace and a feeling of connected-ness. When I am at peace with being alone, I stand connected in my solitude. I no longer perceive others as separate because I know that I am a part of all that exists around and inside of me.

The inevitable physical isolation we experience as CFS patients doesn't have to lead to emotional isolation. Being alone can be a respite and a time of divine connection. It can be a time to reflect, a time to discover new parts of ourselves. Now is our time to leave some of the world behind. It is the season for some aspects of ourselves to die so we can eventually create new meaning and a new self. CFS doesn't just rob us of our very identity, but it brings us to depths of darkness, despair, and isolation that we never would consciously choose—to unveil a new, lighter side of life. Giving up all we once were, we make space to re-create and redefine our selves anew. Much of that creation takes place at times when we are alone, alone to ponder, and alone to wonder. The wondering leads us to new answers and awareness that come only from the physical isolation into which CFS forces us. From darkness into light, our time of lonely isolation emerges into a beautiful time of creation and connection.

GEMS

Isolation is the unwanted feeling of intense lone - liness and alienation, this, accompanied by the belief that you cannot change your reality of separation. The belief, however, is simply that: a belief. All beliefs can be changed.

We all have the opportunity to be a part of the world, because we are a part of it.

One danger of isolation is the bitterness and hopelessness that can follow. The remedy lies in feeling connected and hopeful.

When connecting with people feels too difficult, animals and nature offer a wonderful alternative to isolation.

CFS brings us to the depths of darkness, despair, and isolation to unveil a lighter side of life. When we give up who we once were, we allow ourselves to re-create and re-define ourselves anew.

16
CFS as an Energy Disease

Energy is the seed, the root, the flower of all life. Human energy is a unique thread, woven into the fabric of the universe. When energy is out-of-balance, disease results.

Dr. Edward Taub

About a year ago, after exploring a myriad alternative healing remedies, it occurred to me to once again think metaphorically. It's often easy for me to look at another person's symptom or illness and see a metaphor (a sore throat might represent unspoken or displaced sadness or pain, and a stomachache might signal a distaste for what is going on). When pondering my own CFS, however, I am often mystified. Then one day I had a light bulb moment and this thought illuminated: *Chronic Fatigue Syndrome is an illness characterized by no energy, in other words it is an energetic illness.*

All illness has an energetic component. Illness, words, actions, human beings and all of the universe's creatures are likewise energetic. Everything is energetic. We are as much energy as form.

What does this mean and how does it pertain to CFS?

We typically perceive form/matter and not energy, except in their most obvious manifestations. For instance, it is easy for us to understand that in order for people to function, we need fuel in the form of nutrients, and our level of functioning depends on our energy. This is only one way to see and understand the essence of energy.

Another means of perceiving human energy is our appreciation of what happens when we enter a room full of very angry or sad people. Many of us will enter such an environment and instantly feel the energy, regardless of whether words are exchanged. Here, we are experiencing energy in action.

Energy is everywhere, in everything. We are energy beings. Each thought pondered, each word uttered, and every action taken—all are likewise energy. Energy is reflected by our vitality and our soul. Energy is what connects each one to each other and to the whole.

Through attunement and energy healing, we understand that the energy of one person attracts or repels the energy of another. Each thought, word, and action manifests energetically into our environment and attracts to itself like energy. So, we can imagine a scenario where our energy draws like energy. Let's say, for example, we go into a store while being in a foul mood; perhaps it is not surprising when we have difficulty finding what we are looking for.

We are more powerful as energy beings than as physical beings, God declares in *Conversations With God*. Our thoughts and attitudes are energetically more powerful than what we do. Consider here the power of prayer in healing. Many stories illustrate how ill patients have healed when prayed for.

Viewing Chronic Fatigue Syndrome from this perspective, we understand that this illness manifests energetically as much physically. The physical form consists of all the symptoms we experience. The energetic undercurrent of CFS (the invisible aspects), however includes our thoughts, attitudes, and experiences preceding CFS (the roots beneath the CFS tree), as well as our current reactions to our CFS.

To further appreciate the energetic nature of our CFS, we can practice energy work or visit an energetic healer (someone who offers Reiki, attunement, or healing touch). Or, we can encounter ourselves energetically by going within and gently, lovingly uncovering our thoughts, attitudes, and feelings surrounding our illness. Let me emphasize: this is not to suggest that we brought our CFS upon ourselves; rather, we may want to consider in what ways we have contributed to its development through our mental and emotional energies. Only through honest exploration can we better know ourselves, and give ourselves the opportunity to consciously choose our thought patterns. (To read about and process the power of your thoughts, try Louise Hay's *You Can Heal Your Life* or Walsch's *Conversations With God.*)

When I first encountered the spiritual, energetic healing

art of attunement,* a world of the invisible opened up to me. I learned the experience of energy and developed a new way of understanding the world. Using my hands to feel energy and facilitate its flow, I also learned how to energetically heal others as well as myself. Through my experience of the Divine, I understood that CFS was not only physical, but also energetic.

By this time, I had already unraveled the mystery of CFS intellectually, I knew many of the reasons (thoughts and events) underlying my CFS (refer to the CFS tree illustration)—and most of these were circumstantial and external. Despite having put many of the pieces in place, the mystery puzzle remained incomplete. The missing pieces I had yet to identify were my attitudes and thoughts which lay the foundation and roots of my chronic fatigue.

I realized that my very own attitudes and thoughts shaped the energy of my illness—attitudes of "victim-hood" as a woman in a patriarchal society, thoughts of powerlessness, oppression, and feelings of fear. Initially, these attitudes and thoughts were provoked by my own experience in the dating game, and later, reinforced by theories in psychology and gender classes, and finally realized in my life when I became a victim of male violence (To read about this history, flip to CH: 14, *Uprooting my History.*)

* *Attunement is a spiritual, energy-based healing art developed by vision ary Lloyd Meeker. Using hands (above the body) to guide healing, attunement aligns body, mind, and soul with Divine source by focusing intention and energy on the endocrine glands, organs or specific areas of the body. To learn more, please visit, www.attunement.org*

There are two primary attitudes/feelings that nourished the roots of my CFS; the first of these formed in 1994, while I studied Counseling psychology in graduate school—also marking the beginning of CFS. While at school I worked hard and observed those around me working even harder with jobs, families, and full time school and internships; these thoughts echoed: "This is nuts and hypocritical; how can we be good therapists if we are not being good to ourselves?" I knew deep down that what I saw and what was expected of me were contrary to my soul. Not surprisingly, soon my soul would not let me continue, and after a year in the program, my CFS grew so big I could no longer study.

The second feeling underlying my CFS, another root beneath my CFS tree, was my intensifying fear (between 1992-94), a fear that drew violence into my life. As I read (in psychology) about men abusing women, I became an angry feminist, and soon thereafter what I had read in texts began manifesting in my life. I no longer was merely a victim in my mind, but actually became a victim in life.

We often don't realize the power of our thoughts. Now I do. If we think a thought long and hard enough (even unconsciously), we energetically draw to ourselves that with which we think. In *Conversations With God*, this notion is amplified. God declares: "You call forth precisely what you think, feel, and say."

The energetic undercurrent of my CFS was fear. A fear

that began as a fear of men, and grew into new and different fears over the years until the fears and their invisible energy became physical symptoms. Fear, I have heard, is the most destructive of feelings. It is also something I grappled with daily the year preceding my CFS (via PTSD resulting from a history of violence). Like all emotions good and bad, fear is energetic. Fear destroys, while love heals. We all heal ourselves energetically when we release our negative emotions and thoughts and replace them with positive healing ones.

You might wonder how you can release your negative feelings when they run so deep. You may also question how someone like me, a victim of several violent encounters, could shake her fear and no longer view herself as victim. Truthfully, it has not been easy; I have spent years working to overcome my fears (and continue to do so). Most importantly, I have chosen to surround myself with someone who will support me though the fear. When I find myself in fear of being judged or misunderstood by those around me, I return to those who understand.

In the moment of fear, I try to ask myself if what I am feeling is based on a real present danger or if it is a reaction based on memory and body imprint. When we go through violent traumas, those events are imprinted in our cells and bodies. When a current experience triggers our body memory we may feel the fear all over again whether or not a real danger exists. I can, for example, re-ignite fear when an unexpected loud noise occurs, especially loud voices. Some voices act as triggers for my fears because many of the violent encounters I experienced involved screaming.

When I realize that the danger is not real, I reassure myself over and over that it is imaginary, and take time out to breath deeply. I attempt to reframe what I am experiencing by telling myself a new story. I may, for example, tell myself, "This is not an attack; these voices are normal; you are safe; everything is okay."

My long-term approach to altering my fear has mainly involved my mind. After going through a chain of violent events, I began to think the pattern was just too strong to be mere coincidence. I noted that the violence in my life clearly reflected my fears. I noticed that when I focused on the negative in my mind, my life seemed to reflect that negativity. However, as I grew determined to not only have a better life, but also improve my attitude and thought pattern, my *experience* of life improved. While it took time for my life to "look" the way I envisioned it; I was still able to have a positive experience (much of the time) in the face of whatever life brought me.

Working with the mind and changing our thought patterns is one way to heal ourselves energetically. I personally have found that altering my thoughts from negative to positive can have both short and long-term benefits. When I am feeling particularly down, angry, or frustrated, I first allow myself to experience the feelings. After a time, I decide it is time to move on and will work on my mind to think positively. If I am successful, usually my whole perception changes. For example, when I am down and think about my future and career I frequently believe the future lacks opportunities. After allowing myself to process my feelings and reframe them, however, I can suddenly feel that my future and career look bright.

It is amazing the power our thoughts have on our general outlook. By simply changing our thoughts we can affect profound emotional and physical change—that's energetic healing.

GEMS

Energy is everywhere, in everything. We are energy beings.

The energetic nature of CFS includes our thoughts, attitudes, and experiences preceding CFS (the roots beneath the CFS tree).

When we think long and hard enough, we energetically draw to ourselves that which we think.

17
WHAT HEALS

You will find as you look back upon your life, that the moments that stand out, the moments when you have really lived, are the moments when you have done things in the spirit of love.

Henry Drummond

When the idea for this chapter first emerged I was sure that the content would be treatment-based. *"It'll explain various treatments for the diverse CFS symptoms and imbal-ances,"* I thought. As the words found their way to paper, however, the content evolved into something quite different. *What Heals* is not about treatments, but rather about lifestyle—making healthy choices and taking restorative actions.

When you decide to heal your CFS, you embark on a complex and exciting journey. To help you along the way, I have identified 19 lifestyle actions to aid in your healing. This section begins with a simple explanation of the nature of the CFS healing journey, and follows with practical suggestions for your healing.

For every person with CFS there is a unique story, a unique symptomology, and a unique onset. The same is true for our healing—what works for one person will not necessarily work for another because each body is unique and each symptom constellation different.

Length of CFS

The length of CFS can vary greatly. Some with CFS are fortunate to only experience it for six months to a year (these are the minority), while the rest of us live with it anywhere from a few years up to 20 years, or even life-long. Why this is so can only be conjectured, as there haven't been conclusive studies (to the best of my knowledge) that address the subject. However, we can speculate as to why some people heal more quickly than others. Those who accept their illness, who are determined and believe in their recovery, and who maintain a strong will may be better off than those with pessimistic, victim mentalities. Certainly, many doctors and healers (Bernie Siegel, Andrew Weil, and Louise Hays) have seen the benefits of positive attitudes on their patients.

Healing CFS involves a journey with no quick fixes or "cure-alls" because there is no single identifiable cause leading to one particular treatment. The causes are many; thus healing may best involve addressing the many physical imbalances while simultaneously examining your emotional and mental stressors.

THE HEALING JOURNEY

1. Embrace CFS

To heal CFS, you first need to stop fighting your illness and embrace it. You are taking a journey that involves more than what you can see on the surface. You are healing a weakened body as well as hopefully addressing the underlying parts of yourself that need your attention.

This is your time to let go of agendas and societal commitments, and focus on yourself. You are about to discover some new, exciting, and yes, sometimes frightening insights about yourself. First and foremost, CFS is a time to slow down and learn to accept your present physical, mental, and emotional limitations (and strengths) as best as you can.

2. Decide to Heal

Once you accept that you are indeed ill and on a healing journey requiring patience, love, and trust, it is time to *decide to heal*. Deciding to heal is about deciding you *can* and *will* get better. It is about your will—something CFS cannot take from you unless you choose to give your power away.

When you decide to heal, you have taken a key step on the path to healing. Each treatment you try, and each emotional or mental issue you overcome, becomes a stepping-stone on your way to wellness. Sometimes, though, the stone you have stepped on is not visible (and will not appear until later), leaving you to believe that your actions have done little and helped even less. Remember: everything begins as energy, and however invisible, every action spawns a reaction. No positive action is fruitless.

3. Trust the Healing Process

Trust your healing process. Know that each positive choice you make brings you closer to health. Trust that you are making healthful choices and that seeing improvement is not always your reward. Sometimes our rewards do not manifest physically. Instead, our reward comes from making a change we believe in or learning about a new remedy that helps us feel empowered. The possible rewards are endless and not limited to physical improvement.

Remember: a lot is transpiring, detoxifying and repairing inside of you—most of which you'll never see. We often think when we begin to feel better it is because of something we recently did. Maybe yes, maybe no. How can we know for sure? Perhaps it's a cumulative result of small shifts from all the healing work we've been doing, and now our body is ready to manifest a renewed vigor or improved functioning. Keep this in mind when you feel you're working hard on healing and not experiencing any improvement.

4. Know It Takes Time

Healing CFS takes time. It took time to develop the illness (although you probably didn't experience it that way), and it takes time to heal. Just how much time healing will require is partially up to you and partially up to nature, God, the Divine. However, since you don't really know how long it will take to heal, why not decide for yourself that it won't take too long. Decide such, work toward that goal, and do everything you can to make it so.

5. Decide How Long

You may think that deciding how long it's going to take to heal sounds crazy, but we do it unconsciously all the time. We go to a doctor, ask how long we might have

CFS and the doctor says, "Could be five, ten, 15 years. I don't know." We leave demoralized because we thought we'd be better within a year. So, why change our thinking to match the doctor's when s/he just admitted to not really knowing?

If you have too much faith in your doctor's prolonged diagnosis, your healing just might stretch out over more than a decade when it didn't necessarily have to—and wouldn't that be a hell of a shame? Your doctor doesn't know and maybe you don't either, but what you believe will impact what you experience.

I know my thinking has impacted many aspects of my life. I've also observed others living out their beliefs. Here are two stories of people with CFS, each with opposing beliefs and attitudes. The first is about a man who got CFS while in college. This man, like so many, did much to heal, including authoring a book about his disease, but after 15 years, he still lived a life scarred by CFS. His main response to CFS was to lament it, seeing it as his enemy. Of course, he never knew when he would get better, but chose to believe that he may have CFS for life.

Ten years ago, another college student came down with a mysterious illness that also turned out to be CFS. She, like the man in the first story, becoming debilitated by CFS, had to leave school. Initially, the woman's days were filled with clouds, filled with frustration, distress, and depression. However, after a year or so, she decided to focus on healing and believe that CFS wouldn't be hers for long, and this change renewed her morale.

After three years of wavering determination, she decided, "Enough was enough!" and decided to stop being miserable and focus on getting and feeling better. As the next year progressed, she made healthy choices and began to experience dramatic improvements. Those progressive strides, coupled with her determination to heal, led the student to decide that she would be totally healed within a year, and while her healing journey did not end in a year's time, her health and attitude continued to improve. (The second student portrayed here is me.)

The year described above has since passed and every year my health improves and CFS loosens its grip; but more importantly, every year I grow as a person largely because of CFS.

6. Embrace Optimism

So why do these two people, both with the same disease, experience such divergent journeys? The answer may lie in their different beliefs and attitudes about this illness (namely, how long their CFS will endure, how much they can do about it, and how they feel about their CFS.) Being optimistic or thinking positively has both emotional and physical rewards. Emotionally, optimism feeds the heart and soul and makes a person feel good in spite of it all. Physically, optimism feeds the immune system, strengthening it.

7. Be Response-able

This brings me to the next key ingredient to healing: your attitude. What you think about CFS will influence and sometimes determine what you feel (some will say entirely, but they're ignoring biochemical reactions resulting from physical imbalances). And what you feel will undoubtedly impact your ability to heal. To heal, you'll need a large dose of *optimism*. It helps if you can see that there are benefits (as well as pitfalls) to CFS. It also helps if you choose to be responsible for your healing without carrying the burden of self-blame for acquiring CFS in the first place.

Some people take the notion of self-responsibility too far, claiming that empowered beings choose their destinies. If you are feeling overwhelmed by the notion that you may have caused your illness or that you should make yourself better, let go. Let all those negative, self-defeating thoughts go. You have inadvertently taken the "self-responsibility" concept too far and this will not serve you. We *can* do a lot to heal and we are empowered beings. In fact, we're our own best healers, but we also need help. Nobody does anything completely alone. Look for help, get it, and believe in yourself without the blaming. CFS is a gift that entered your life to make it better; while that may not be apparent, eventually the reasons for your CFS will unfold.

8. Have Patience

Be patient. All is well. Your healing will come. Being patient means riding through the difficult times and trusting that the end is in sight. Patience means allowing the healing process to unfold while doing what you can to help it along: exercising; eating healthy foods; addressing yeast and digestive problems; cleansing yourself and your environment; getting adequate sunlight, air, and contact with nature; doing the things you love—whatever they may be; making sure your life has meaning and humor; and surrounding yourself with supportive people.

9. Act From the Heart

How do you decide what to do to heal?

There are plenty of CFS books (many of which are wonderful) filled with all kinds of treatment alternatives: "What to do if so-and-so ails you." Go ahead and find at least one book you would like to use as a reference, a guidepost. Then, use yourself. Pay attention to how you feel, to where things are coming from, and then, to the best of your ability, address each one. Try only treatments that feel "right." If you honestly don't believe something will work, don't bother, but make sure you talk this decision over with your healer. If you don't trust or like your doctor or healer, find another.

You are your own best guide. Let your body, your experience, your intuition, and your heart guide your choice of action. Choose only what feels good or make an attitudinal shift to feel good about what you believe will work. It will be difficult, yes, but worth it.

Had you told me a year ago that I would rarely drink or crave coffee, I would have argued with you. After gradually eliminating my beloved java, first by switching to decaffeinated coffee, then weaning myself off that, I cleansed my body of its addiction. I became even more determined to give up other less-than-positive behaviors when I began to experience amazing physical improvements.

We can do a lot once we make up our minds and finally go for it. We can learn to love something we once hated, even giving up our favorite food and/or vice.

10. Do What You Love

If you don't love what you are doing, than decide to do only what you love. I am not talking here so much about what CFS treatments you choose, (although the idea is applicable there as well). I am referring here to what you do when you're not working to heal your CFS.

A lot of people hate their jobs. That causes a lot of unhealthy, unnecessary stress. If that's your case, try to find another job, or at the very least find some things about your job that you do like. Focus your thoughts on what is working in your life, not what isn't. Where we invest our energy speaks to what we attract energetically; so invest it in loving what you do. When you love what you do, life is easier, less stressful, and you feel good about yourself. And good feelings heal.

11. Treat Yourself

Whenever I have a challenge in my life, I like to give myself an incentive by attaching a reward to my facing up to it. For example, if I have to study for an exam, I'll tell myself that if I study for three hours, I will treat myself to a movie or something equally enjoyable.

Life is meant to be joy-full, but most of us neglect to reward ourselves for our efforts. CFS usually feels more like struggle than reward, so it's important to turn this adversity into pleasantry as much as possible. You can do this by rewarding yourself with activities you love, small gifts to yourself, affirmations that honestly declare just how great you are. Rewards don't need to be limited to material objects, they can also come via simple activities, such as listening to your favorite music, picking a flower, calling a good friend, or soaking in a hot bath. When you treat yourself, you are healing your CFS through good feelings and helpful chemical reactions.

12. Change Your Diet

Some people with heart conditions ignore medical advice and refuse to change their eating habits; some may refuse to give up favorite foods—even at the expense of their very lives. Why? I know exactly why. Giving up our beloved treats seems like yet another loss in a long list of them. "What's the point of living," they may think; "if I have to give up everything I love about my life?" Of course, if you only focus on what you're "losing," you perceive it as losing. What if you knew that giving up sugar, for example, would lead to a 75-percent increase in daily energy. Wouldn't you do it?

The catch here is that there are no guarantees of improved health for the heart patient, and he knows it. He may rather spend his last days enjoying the pleasures of his unhealthy foods than give them up, on the chance that he may increase his life span.

There are no guarantees. I can't guarantee that if you

make significant dietary changes you'll feel better, but I can promise that your body will perform better in the long run.

As explained in the CH 27: *Nourish Thy Body*, most American diets are high in sugar, fat, and toxins. If you're someone with this diet, your immune system is suffering, and so are your digestive and nervous systems. Eating a diet high in: fat, sugar, meat proteins, caffeine, and refined, processed foods, and replacing it with one high in: whole fruits, vegetables, legumes, grains, and healthy proteins will help you heal in two ways. First, you'll be providing your already compromised body with nourishing fuel. And second, you will not be adding foods that are difficult to digest or toxins that your body must work to eliminate (which only exacerbate your symptoms and problems).

People often say "bad foods" taste so good, but I've discovered that healthy foods taste far better, and I am boosted by the added confidence of knowing I am being a healthier person. When you eat "junk food," there may be a part of your consciousness that feels shame or regret. Why create an internal battle in your mind or body? Choose foods consciously, eat healthy, and enjoy your meals.

13. Live Stress free

It's likely that stress played a role in your CFS. Now it's time to de-stress. This can be challenging in a fast-paced, "do-do" society, but with CFS, it's almost a natural consequence. You just can't keep up the stress-filled life; so it's best if you just leave it behind. Stress is not a necessary component in our lives; we merely created the myth that it is. CFS teaches us to return to our stress-free, carefree, relaxed nature. As we eliminate stress, we likewise eliminate many challenges to our body, and that's what healing is all about.

14. Create Meaning

Most of us will (at some juncture in our lives) ask ourselves, "Why am I here?" Maybe you'll fall into an identity crisis as you struggle with the losses created by CFS. I sure did.

When everything was black and bleak, I began asking myself scary, yet important questions: *"What is my purpose?"* Somehow, CFS led me not only to the question, but to my answers as well. Along the way, I discovered a vital aspect to any life—meaning.

If there is no meaning, there is emptiness; it is a kind of nothingness that makes healing impossible. Purpose motivates, inspires, and directs us. Having purpose or meaning in your life invigorates the body and soul. If you're unclear about this aspect of your life, make it a part of your healing journey to search, explore, and discover the true meaning of your life.

15. Discover The Humor

To the CFSer, events often feel larger than life and we may over-react to our difficult circumstances and chemical imbalances, making mountains out of molehills. It can feel (at times) as if everything is "life or death." Despite this perception, nothing is so serious that you can't find humor in it.

CFS can trick us into becoming glum, down-in-the-dumps people. If you ever watch Jay Leno on the *Tonight*

Show, you'll see a man who makes fun of everyone and everything, himself included. His point—and mine—is don't take it all so seriously. Enjoy life. Find time to play with reckless abandon. Laugh at your getting lost in the parking lot. Giggle at your inability to remember a name or word. Find humor in the insane; that's what humor is for—showing us the absurdity in what we experience.

Anything can appear hilarious if presented and perceived that way. Rent funny movies, read stupid joke books, share silly stories, and delight in the absolute absurdity of CFS. Sometimes CFS is just plain funny, and laughter is consistently proven to be a great medicine. (Norman Cousins, in *Anatomy of an Illness*, speaks to this.)

16. Delight in the Great Outdoors

God is at his most spectacular in nature. The place to recognize pure perfection and the beauty of it all is in nature. Part of nature includes our body and its complex healing process, but nature is also everything else outside our front door (if it's not paved over!).

Go outside. Be with the beauty. Get some sunlight. Remember from whence you came. See the perfection you miss when you live a busy life. Acknowledge the gift CFS gives you, the gift of enjoying what God created for you, me, and everyone. Enjoy the animals, soil, sky, hills, mountains, and the trees. Smell the wafting sea breezes, the scent of pines, blooming flowers, or whatever is alive right now, right outside your door. Every time you appreciate nature, you give yourself the gift of healing.

17. Get Exercise

Mobile people mobilize their cells through the oxygen they breath. Deep, slow breathing accompanied by muscle movement is not only healing to the body, but also does wonders for the soul. I find that walking, dancing, and yoga—whatever physical action I am capable of—frees my pent-up energies and feels immensely therapeutic.

Our bodies were meant to move. For people with CFS, moving becomes difficult especially since physical exertion is frequently followed by fatigue and increased symptoms. Yet, on the other hand, a lack of movement can also set us back. Finding our capacity to exercise can be a trial-and-error process. Sometimes you have to "overdo it" a few times before you fully understand what works and what doesn't. You can simply start with walking, stretching, or practicing basic yoga. (A great book about the healing power of yoga is Agombar's *Beat Fatigue with Yoga*.)

As you strengthen your immune system, lungs, and muscles, you can increase duration or add new activities to your routine. Keep it slow but steady, like CFS itself. After a time, your improved well-being will give you the incentive to keep it up. It's wonderful to experience continued physical improvement through increased activity, but it is also important to be aware that a common CFS side effect to exercise is increased fatigue and symptoms. This is especially true after aerobic activity. So, it is critical that CFSers begin exercising slowly and preferably choose non-aerobic activities to start.

Personally, I found I could ease into yoga and do it even when exhausted. I began by following the yoga routines in Lark's *Chronic Fatigue and Tiredness*. Eventually, I bought a video and tried Ashtanga yoga, at my doctor's advice. I also tried classes and continue to regularly practice yoga on my own. I've learned along the way, after only a few minutes of yoga I can transform exhaustion into rejuvenation.

18. Spend Time Among Friends

We all need support, support in our treatment, support during stressful times, and support on our healing journey. Support will not come from everyone. In fact, you may find support is sorely lacking in ways you believe you need it most.

I talk a lot about support in the form of relationship in the chapters 21, 22, and 15: *Relationships and CFS, The CFS Couple,* and *Inevitable Isolation.* Here, I wish to introduce a new element. We can derive support from people in all arenas of life. If we aren't finding it in our core relationships, than maybe we can get it from unexpected sources. For example, a teacher may give you extra time to finish a paper because you confided in him about your CFS. Or, when you tell a stranger on an airplane about CFS, maybe for the first time you feel heard and supported. Whatever the circumstance, there will always be people in our lives who challenge us, and those who are our angels, helping and supporting us. Notice the latter. Thank them. Seek out more like them. People can help you feel your CFS is not only manageable, but even miraculous.

If you have difficulty finding "live" people to support

you, consider an Internet chat room for CFSers or watch movies that lend support. One of my best supports is the *Oprah* Show. Watching her uplifting show helps me feel connected and supported. As I cry during the show, I release feelings that need expression, and so often the stories on the show inspire me eliciting hope.

19. Embrace Faith and Spirit

What you believe, you will see.

Faith is perhaps the biggest influence on your healing and most helpful to your soul. If you believe in some greater "something"—God, the Divine, Source, Higher Being, however you wish to define *It*—you give yourself immense support. Prayer, faith, and trust give you strength when you're down, and provide direction when you lack one.

It wasn't until CFS that I discovered my true connection to the Divine. I had always thought of myself as a spiritual person but never really lived out my spiritual values. Then one day, I realized my connection to spirit. I learned the beautiful healing/energetic art of attunement and it gave me a newfound awareness of the power in the invisible. Through it, I learned to sense divinity all around me. I let it heal me. With my hands, my heart, and my openness, I "attuned" myself when I was down, when I was exhausted, when I had a headache, and when cramps came. Many times, after only a few minutes of attunement, my pain vanished, energy flowed and mood improved. These transformations gave me a real sense of awe in the unseen, in the Divinity, and in myself.

One day, as I was going about my usual day, which was not very usual, I heard a voice within declare: "read *Conversations With God.*" That voice led me to pick the book up, and I was instantly hooked. A year prior, I had seen the book at Barnes and Noble and scoffed at its title. "Who does this guy think he is?" I mused, reacting to the author's gall at announcing himself as communicating with God. But in spite of my initial judgment, I later devoured the first book, then the second, and soon the third.

Through my spiritual feast that came via these books, I experienced renewal, belief, and optimism. Suddenly, spirituality was no longer merely a concept, but my way of perceiving and being. As my connection to Divine spirit grew, my health improved. And, then I knew there was more than what could be seen with one's eyes, and I knew that that-which-could-not-be-seen loved and supported me.

Find your truth. Nourish your wisdom. Resurrect your faith and create spirituality. Affirm through prayer and gratitude. Prayer heals. Faith heals. Having spirit in your life will give you the support you need when you cannot find it elsewhere.

GEMS

19 Ways to Heal CFS

1. embrace CFS
2. decide to heal
3. trust the healing process
4. know it takes time
5. decide how long
6. embrace optimism
7. be response-able
8. have patience
9. act from the heart
10. do what you love
11. treat yourself
12. change your diet
13. live stress-free
14. create meaning
15. discover the humor
16. delight in the great outdoors
17. get exercise
18. spend time among friends
19. embrace faith

18
YOU ARE YOUR OWN BEST HEALER

Like most people in our society, I grew up believing in the medical myth. I grew up believing that health comes from the doctor, the drug store, and the hospital. I never suspected that illness might be a messenger, or that our experience of our bodies, whether well or ill, could provide us with self-understanding. I never imagined that the source of true healing lay within each of us...

John Robbins

Last night I was inspired and tickled by one doctor's extraordinary attitude toward medicine when I saw the movie *Patch Adams*. Patch is not the only doctor out there who cares about his patients, but he is one of the rare ones who will consider the person before the disease. There are other greats like him, thank goodness. I've also been inspired by the work and words of Norman Cousins, Bernie Siegel, and Andrew Weil. These doctors believe in the patient, in quality of life, and believe in the innate healing power of every human being. Luckily for me, my family doctor seems to share these beliefs.

Your body is meant to be healthy. Its natural state is one of good health. Your current state of ill health is your body's unnatural state. Your body, with your help, is trying to return to homeostasis, balance—health.

If your experience is like mine, a part of you is saying, "If I just knew exactly what was wrong, then I could (or my doctor could) find the perfect treatment and I would get healthy again." Or, perhaps you're thinking, "If only I could find a good doctor, than I could get better." Or how about this one, "If only I had enough money to cover the costs of this treatment, than I could get better."

In any case, if you are thinking such thoughts, you are essentially doing the same thing. You are creating the belief that your healing is dependent on something *outside* yourself and is not within your reach. You are seeing yourself as a victim of an illness that cannot be healed because certain conditions necessary for your healing are not available. You are a victim of your own creation, because you have made yourself powerless despite your good intentions to the contrary. Someone else or something else is the powerful one—the doctor, the elusive, mystery treatment—someone or something besides you.

We all think this way at one time or another. I certainly have played the victim, and have gotten caught in thinking, "If only..." The truth is doctors may help you, but you must help yourself, too. How do I know this to be true? I can look at my own healing and see that my doctors have helped me (most of all with their caring and openness), but their help has only contributed to part of my healing.

A larger healing has come about from me: my choices, my beliefs, my actions, and my dedication and determination to heal. If you look at the history of Chronic Fatigue Syndrome, you will see a disease that has continually baffled and frustrated the entire medical establishment; those in it have been unable to identify the cause, or find a reliable treatment, or "cure." In fact, most of the doctors I consulted early on were un-able to tell me anything about CFS beyond what I already knew: "Take care of yourself, get rest, and avoid stress," they would say.

Unfortunately, some medical professionals, feeling powerless when faced with CFS and driven to do something, anything, will prescribe antidepressants. In some cases, this prescription might make sense,* but when they were prescribed to me, I knew the doctor was lost. Scribbling the prescription on his tablet, he handed it to me and requested I come back in a year! This same doctor ridiculed me when he saw pigment loss on my chest during the examination, and belittled me for questions regarding the CFS studies I had read. He was by far the worst doctor I have ever seen, but the embodiment of what I'm talking about—a doctor who feels the need to be the expert and in control, yet has very little to offer except condescension and pat non-responses. Ironically, his name was listed in a city medical directory as a CFS Specialist—some specialist! So beware, sometimes doctors do more harm than good.

* According to Kenny (94), antidepressants are frequently prescribed to CFSers in minute doses (about 1/10th that of what a depressed person receives) to correct an imbalance in the brain's serotonin levels.

More recently, however I have encountered doctors who are compassionate and knowledgeable about CFS. Still, the fact remains that CFS is not *fully* understood by anyone including doctors in the medical community. Therefore, CFS requires doctors and patients alike to explore new paths, new theories, and new treatments. I think that CFS, in particular, calls upon doctors to treat each patient individually.

CFS is just one of many contemporary illnesses that demonstrates the multi-dimensional nature of our beings and the need to heal holistically. Environmental-related and immune deficiency diseases (e.g., Gulf-war Syndrome, multi-chemical sensitivities, lupus...) also speak to the need for people to be in balance within themselves and in harmony with the planet. Our health depends upon much more than healthy bodies, but also healthy minds, spirit, and a healthy environment.

The problem with going to a doctor to help you "cure" CFS is that your physician most likely views only one dimension of you—your body. CFS is an illness that requires looking at much more—your mind, emotions, the environment around you, and your spirit as well. (I would argue, in fact, that this is true of all maladies, but I think it is especially true about CFS.) Besides the fact that your doctor will not likely take into consideration the realms of mind and spirit (unless you are lucky enough to have a holistic-minded doctor like mine), nor encourage you to do so; they may have less expertise than they think. Sure, maybe they have studied the human body and physiology for years, even decades, but is this doctor *inside* your body, living out your experience?

No doctor can be you, feeling CFS on a daily basis. Without you, what your doctor knows has little meaning unless they can use it to help you heal. I think doctors forget this, and fail to give their patients due credit. You know what's going on inside of you better than anyone—and that alone is powerful! You are closer to the source of the problem than anyone. Your doctor may not give you credit for your knowledge, but then you probably don't give yourself much credit either. You are so much more than you give yourself credit for, especially when it comes to your healing ability.

How can you be so critical of your ability to heal when you hold the key? The most important aspect of your healing is something only you can control—your attitude. How you feel and what you think about your CFS, affect not only your healing but also your experience of your illness. Only *you* experience the pain and symptoms of CFS. Only *you* experience your disparaging thoughts, feelings of sadness, anger, frustration, and hopelessness. Only *you* can make the effort and commitment to follow treatments, take prescriptions, and change your diet. Only *you* can *do* what is necessary to heal. Only *you* can change these thoughts and attitudes.

Andrew Weil addresses the effects of attitude on healing in his wonderful book *Spontaneous Healing*. In it, he identifies acceptance as the single most important aspect in healing. He also notes the powerful innate capacity of the body to heal itself, and explains how eventually bodies do heal themselves. Of course, we can help that innate healing along by changing our attitude toward our illness. If we focus our energy on the positive aspects of our lives, including what our illness may teach us, we will have done a great deal to move ourselves toward healing.

GEMS

You see yourself as a victim of CFS when you believe yourself powerless, seeing your doctor or some mystery treatment as all-powerful. Doctors can help, but you must be the key player in your healing.

What heals your CFS: are your choices, beliefs, actions, dedication and determination to heal. That's what heals.

The most important aspect of your healing journey is what you control, your attitude.

19
GRATITUDE FOR THE GIFT

Healing is the process of accepting all, then choosing best.

Neale Donald Waslch

If you haven't reached a place where you can imagine anything beneficial from CFS then it will be virtually impossible for you to feel grateful for your illness. Knowing that CFS has something to offer you is its gift to you. CFS is a gift to awaken your lost soul.

The hardest, darkest time of my experience with Chronic Fatigue Syndrome came at a time I grappled with questions of self-identity; *Who am I? What is my purpose? Why am I here?* In those dark hours, my only answers were equally dark: "You have no purpose, no reason to be here," I heard myself respond. Those times were scary, far more desolate than any CFS symptoms I have experienced. And yet, those questions were necessary. CFS led me to those questions, questions to awaken my soul, questions to begin the soul-searching aspect of my *Call For Soulwork.*

Every illness arrives in our lives as a driving force; their purpose not to give us pain, confusion, or a sore throat, but rather to help us. Our symptoms are mere circumstances in our reality; they are not our soulwork. Beneath the symptoms lay purpose—the purpose: *our soulwork*. It is our time to explore our depths. It is time to define, re-define, and recreate who we believe ourselves to be. Who we are is not our illness, although our illness can help us to understand who we are.

When you are able to see the beauty in moving beyond symptoms to discover their purpose, you will discover the gift of CFS. Receive your gift; feel grateful. Feel grateful and act from that place of being.

You may ask, *How can I show my gratitude for CFS? To whom shall I be grateful?* We can be grateful for the experience and give something to the universe in return—expressing our thanks via our attitudes, love and appreciation. When we speak of or write about gratitude we increase positive feelings and help ourselves to heal.

Through every thought of gratitude, I release chemicals into my body that strengthen my immune system, heart, and cells. Gratitude is a feeling that both lightens and enlightens my being. It helps me to see the beauty in the absurd and the joy in adversity.

When I feel grateful for one area in my life, other things I am grateful for spring forth. The mere act of expressing gratitude seems to bring about more gratitude. It is like seeing one wave and then suddenly realizing it is part of a vast ocean. When I can find one thing about CFS that I am grateful for, I discover a wealth of additional things to feel grateful for, and the net-effect is I feel better and transform into a better person.

In the thick of CFS symptoms, I often struggle to see what it has given me. Hopefully, as I share with you what I have realized to be the gifts of my CFS, you too will be inspired to recognize yours.

CFS has truly given me a lot of amazing gifts. It has helped me to know that I am not what I do. I am beautiful just as I am. I need not prove myself. CFS has returned me to creativity. It has helped me appreciate not only relationships with family and friends, but relationships in general, with strangers, with people in public services, and my healers. CFS has helped me realize that it does not matter from whom I receive love, so long as it is there. It has brought the world of animals ever so big into my heart especially when the world of people has felt intimidating, too demanding, or loud. The healing process has led me to the experience of attunement and to God. CFS has truly blessed me.

CFS has also led me to learn about countless healing arts and remedies, about human anatomy, aromatherapy, herbology, nutrition, and Ayurvedic medicine. It has shown me that I am both teacher and student. It has highlighted my addictions to sugar and caffeine and helped me to overcome these. It has increased my awareness on so many levels inspiring me to share ideas, to write and teach about them.

I hope that my *Call For Soulwork* will help you, and in so doing, we are both blessed by CFS. Thank you, CFS. Thank you, God.

GEMS

Every illness arrives in our lives as a driving force; their purpose not to give us pain, confusion, sore throats, but rather to help us.

Beneath the symptoms lay purpose, our Soulwork. Soulwork is our time to explore our depths.

Who we are is not our illness, but our illness can help us to understand who we are.

20
BEFRIENDING THE PAIN

A warrior doesn't seek pain, but if pain comes, he uses it.

Dan Millman

Pain results from a judgment you have made about a thing. Remove the judgment and the pain disappears.

Neale Donald Walsch

As I learned to let go of my grievances through the practice of forgiveness, my pain disappeared.

Gerald Jampolsky

Pain, like many other symptoms of CFS, exists so as to call our awareness to a specific area of our lives or perhaps to an area in our body that needs attention. Pain screams out, literally clamoring for your attention.

When pain calls, listen. Listen carefully. Pain is likely the most difficult of symptoms to embrace because we've been taught, "Have a headache? Take this. Heartburn a problem? Take that. Excruciating stomachache? Take this and that." It's always the same message: *don't let pain stand in the way, eradicate it with a pill.* It's as if pain is the ultimate enemy with no purpose other than to annoy, distract, and hurt.

The truth is the media and society have got it backwards.

Don't nullify and anesthetize your pain; pay attention to it. Say, "Hello!" and converse with it. Embrace your pain. Your pain wants your attention. Have you ever truly sat with it, not wishing it away or condemning it, but welcoming it as a teacher? Yes, a teacher: an entity that has something helpful and important to say.

The first step in hearing a message is to receive the messenger. As hard as it may be, focus all of your attention on the place of your pain. (Perhaps you should only try this if your pain is not debilitating or not affecting your entire body.) I recommend people befriend their pain early on in the process, preferably at its onset, and try this exercise only when it feels do-able.

Now, breathe into it. Journey into its center, taking deep inhalations and long, slow exhalations. Notice everything. *How much does it hurt? What other sensations and thoughts are you having?* Stay with your pain and experience it to its depths. Try asking the pain (or where it hurts) questions; ask with love, receive with openness. Anticipate nothing. Relinquish this moment to your pain. Let pain be your guide and friend.

If conversations don't come easily, you may wish to try drawing your pain or writing down your dialogue. For example, you could begin by asking: *Pain, why are you here?* Then ask, *what is it you wish to tell me?*

Sometimes, it's not possible to befriend pain, because the pain has taken over completely. Perhaps in this case, taking a pain reliever is indeed the best response. Or, maybe taking a warm bath, getting a massage, energy work, or acupuncture will help relieve the pain and enable you to relax. Whatever you do, choose something relaxing. Pain increases in stress and low-oxygen states. So whatever you do, try to reduce stress and breath deeply.

Perhaps all these ideas seem foreign to you because your pain is so constant, so debilitating. Have you only allowed pain to be your enemy? If that's the case, ask yourself: *Have I done everything in my power to shun and destroy it, as if it truly were an archenemy to be defeated?* I suggest that at some time you consider a new approach. Try adopting love instead of fear, and embracing your pain instead of eradicating it.

Throughout my teens and twenties, pain was a monthly occurrence. It came every period and was relentless. Once, when I was rocking up and down, cradling myself in the midst of crippling cramps, I tried accepting and embracing my pain.

After years of believing pain to be the enemy and attempting whatever was necessary to rid myself of it, I finally decided to try a different approach. Previously, I had always embraced the attitude most pervasive in our society: pain is bad, the enemy. My only objective was to conquer it by getting rid of it. But, years spent waging war with pain had taught me nothing. The pain was always the victor, coming back again and again as if to say, "Gretchen, I am here and you better deal with me this time." Funny thing was I never really let myself just "hang out" with it. So, one day, that's exactly what I decided to do. What did I have to lose? Nothing else worked.

So, I did exactly what I am recommending you do. I breathed into my pain. I yielded to it by entering it; and to my amazement, my encounter was both moving and trans-formative. The more I stayed with the pain, put my awareness deep into it, the more I felt the pain give way. I noticed too that the pain had rhythm; it changed color. It was even possible to feel the pain as strong and persistent, yet notice that the more I maintained my attention on the intensity, the actual pain of the feelings dissipated. I imagine this type of experience: simultaneous intense sensations coupled with a decrease in pain, may be similar to what some moth-ers feel during childbirth. Contrary to our understanding, it's possible to feel immense pain, but not be in-pain.

I share my story not to emphasize a result, but rather to illustrate the unproductive nature of treating pain as "bad." *Do you really want to be at war with your own body?* Pain is in your body and therefore part of it. Declaring war on your body cannot possibly be anything but destructive. You have other choices. You always do.

You don't have to see your pain as the enemy. You can learn to befriend your pain and gain tremendous insight when not opposing it. You can breathe into it, dialogue with it, draw it, massage it, bathe it, do energy work with it, dance with it, or you can beat a drum to its pulse. You can

196

interact with your pain in countless ways.

Most of the suggestions here are free and will help set you free. If you have only tried nullifying your pain, try another path, the path of least resistance: friendship. Befriending your pain is like forgiving your enemy. It releases you and frees you. All your energy once engaged in fight is now available for healing.

Have you heard anything but miraculous stories regarding the power of forgiveness? Forgiveness and the act of befriending are twins. They function the same way. When you forgive someone, you give yourself the gift of love by opening your heart and in the process you are set free. *Forgiveness is about you, not about who you forgive.* The same holds true with befriending your pain. When you finally stop resisting and start embracing your pain, you free up a lot of energy that has been pent-up in fighting mode, and you free yourself from an inner war—where the only loser is you.

This is the first blessing. Your second blessing comes when you uncover the message underlying the pain. And trust me, it is there waiting to be found. When the pain leads you on a path to new awareness, you will truly under-stand the meaning and reason for befriending it.

Until I reached my thirties, I had spent a lot of energy rejecting a part of myself. Each time my period arrived, I dreaded it because it always brought excruciating pain, uncontrollable emotions, and frequent bouts of sickness.

Early on, I learned to reject my cycle by trying not to think about it; and when it came, I took ibuprofen hoping to nullify it. Also whenever the pain arrived, I grew fearful. At the first hint of pain, I only anticipated difficulty and suffering. My attitude toward my cycle was one filled with fear and trepidation.

There were additional ways I rejected my feminine side. After years of male harassment followed by numerous violent attacks by men, I began to associate my sexuality with these events. As a means of protection, I learned yet again to reject a part of my femininity. Unfortunately, the side effects were costly: I lost my sex-drive and intimacy with my husband. (I often wonder how much of this history has contributed to my hormonal imbalances.)

My intense fear of both pain and violence taught me rejection and constriction. And the pain did not relent until I learned another approach. Rather than continuing my fearful reaction and fight with pain, I learned to work with it. When it arrived, I would try very hard not to fear it (it often requires a lot of effort to change personal programming), and instead I would try breathing deeply into it, asking Carl to help me, by applying pressure to my lower back at the same time. Other times, I would apply attunement, using my hands energetically with the pain, and as I did, my fear of pain decreased. Over time, the pain also diminished.

Through the process of engaging rather than fearing my pain, I decreased my judgments of it. Instead, I learned to let pain be. And as I let it be, my pain freed me to see that it, in and of itself, is not the enemy.

I continue from time to time to experience pain. Now, when pain comes, I try to remember it is my teacher— always telling me to slow down, breath, not to worry, and to be in the here and now. Time and again, pain reminds me of my feminine side and how it needs expression; and it reminds me to *be* when I get overly driven into *doing*.

There are cycles to a body's rhythm that mirror that of the planet, the tides, and moon. Cycles, like waves, cannot be controlled. Nor should they be. Part of femininity, I have learned, is to trust these cycles, the rhythms that connect to nature and all that is. This is what my pain helps me remember.

Your pain may have a different message. Try to listen.

GEMS

Pain, like so many other symptoms, asks us to become aware of something in our lives. Try adopting love with pain instead of fear; embrace your pain instead of eradicating it.

Learn to befriend your pain and gain tremendous insight when not opposing it. You can breath into it, dialogue with it, draw it, massage it, bathe it, do energy work with it, dance with it, or beat a drum to its pulse.

21
THE CFS COUPLE

When you own what you feel, you are empowered to make conscious choices about how to change the feeling. When other people know what you feel, you are empowered to both create and define boundaries.

Iyanla Vanzant

When a couple is faced with CFS, the relationship invariably changes, and at first glance, not in positive ways. The best way to handle this disruption is to acknowledge it with compassion and to discuss its impact together as a couple.

Carl and I learned the hard way. Nine years after CFS had made its way into every facet of our relationship, we finally sat down to discuss what CFS meant. Somehow, getting caught up in the day-to-day of it, we had never taken the time to discuss what CFS meant to our relationship. Instead, we did what so many other people do: we got married, moved in together, and started our lives together without ever examining how CFS was impacting us. Failing to acknowledge CFS and its role in our lives, we also failed to examine its impact on our future.

At times, CFS overwhelmed both of us. It affected how I felt (helpless and incompetent), how little we could communicate, and how lonely and depressed I had become. CFS altered our relationship and who I had become. Yet in spite of its toll, somehow Carl and I neglected to talk about it. Instead, we lived out our lives unconsciously, falling into roles that neither one of us chose, and eventually leading to our individual frustration and resentment.

There is another way! Now, Carl and I are beginning to dialogue about CFS and its impact on our lives. We are reflecting on powerful questions that should have been addressed when we got engaged, and we are attempting to identify the frustrations and resentments and unravel the tangled mess we got ourselves into. It is hard work, but worthwhile and necessary.

In mere weeks, our relationship has strengthened and we are beginning to rebuild much of the trust lost due to years of poor communication and lack of understanding.

The key to avoiding this kind of pain is strong communication. With your partner, find time to create a loving, accepting environment where the two of you can explore your feelings toward CFS. Consider what you expect from it and each other, and contemplate its impact on *all* of the relationship. Make sure to include a discussion of CFS' impact on **communication, intimacy, money/finances, housework/daily chores,** and **security**. Allow each person time to share without interruption. Decide ahead of time that neither of you will blame one another or fall into the trap of "being right." This is your time for compassionate communication, love, and understanding.

Before discussing these concepts, you may first want to journal to clarify and understand your own feelings. Ask yourself: *What does CFS mean to me and my relationship? What do I want my partner to understand about my CFS? How can my partner assist me? What can my partner and I both do to acknowledge CFS and feel acknowledged?*

Now, look at CFS' impact on the many areas of your relationship. For each of these topics, ask yourself what is important and how CFS has changed that. Ask yourself: *"How does CFS impact my ability to* **communicate** *and be heard? What do I need to better communicate?"*

You may need to agree that when you are dead tired and non-communicative, that you will have some signal to indicate this. Or, you may want to write each other notes during the times when speaking feels daunting or is impossible.

Ask yourself how CFS impacts your **intimacy**. *Have you lost your sex drive? Do you feel that you would rather spend the little energy you have on other activities? Does it change how you express your love and affection? How do the changes in the CFSer impact the partner?*

Consider CFS' impact on **money** and **finances**. *Has CFS robbed you of your ability to work, or has it meant a decreased income? How do you pay for medical expenses? Are you both paying for treatments out-of-pocket? If you* *have insurance, who files the claims? How has CFS altered your financial freedom?*

How has CFS impacted **housework**? *How much does the state of the home affect you both? Who is expected to keep the house clean and organized? How much acknowl - edgement does the housekeeper receive? How can you get the housework done without overly compromising?*

When CFS alters finances, security is shaken. *What does* **security** *mean to you and your partner? How does CFS alter your feelings of security?*

These are just some of the questions you may want to consider. The key here is to acknowledge CFS' impact and examine how it has changed the relationship and your roles within it. You may want to start the conversation by con- templating your roles within the relationship before and after CFS. Try to get to the heart of what you believe and how you feel.

If you are unable to communicate compassionately with your partner about CFS' role within your relationship, seek out a compassionate counselor who can help you address some of these areas. These conversations will trans- form your current relationship as well as your feelings toward one another. Talking openly will help bring you closer together and will facilitate further understanding of one another's needs and feelings surrounding CFS in both of your lives.

GEMS

CFS impacts every aspect of your relationship. The best way to handle this disruption is to acknowledge it.

The key to avoiding pain in your marriage is compassionate communication.

In a journal ask yourself: What does CFS mean to my relationship and me?

With your partner, discuss CFS' impact on:
- *Communication*
- *Intimacy*
- *Money/Finances*
- *Housework/Daily Chores*
- *Security*

22
RELATIONSHIPS & CFS

You will find as you look back upon your life, that the moments that stand out, the moments when you have really lived, are the moments when you have done things in the spirit of love.

Henry Drummond

This chapter came to me many years ago when my CFS was at its worst and I was both physically and emotionally distant from my family. It speaks of a painful time when I felt very alone with CFS. The many bleak descriptions here of my relationships with family and friends have since grown and changed in positive ways.

Knowing of these changes may bring you hope; not only can our relationships with family bring pain, but they may offer healing as well.

This chapter is by far the scariest to share because I fear my family member's reactions. And yet, I am committed to voicing my truth in the hopes that it helps some readers, and I am hopeful that when my family reads this, we will all feel encouraged to dialogue openly about these experiences and everyone's feelings.

I dedicate this chapter to those of you who are alone

in your CFS, for you who struggle with family, and you who need to know where to go for support and help.

If it's not our work that defines who we are, than it's our relationships. Relationships give our lives meaning, direction, love, companionship, and a whole lot more. From within a partnership, a parent-child connection, or a friendship, we share of ourselves and in turn, we receive the love from others. Give and Take. Radiate and receive.

Close relationships often involve a sharing of trust, love, communication, and a cycle of giving and receiving. In healthy relationships, each person gives and receives energy from the relationship not always in equal amounts, but always in a way that facilitates both people feeling cared for.

When one person in the relationship falls ill, the relationship changes. Its give and take nature shifts, and there is likely less equality in the sharing. When a parent, friend, or loved one becomes seriously ill with CFS, they can no longer bring to that relationship what they once did. Instead, the healthier of the two may take on the role of "caretaker." This will inevitably affect the dynamic within the relationship. If perchance this doesn't occur, the ill person may be less involved with their friend/partner because they are preoccupied with, and even handicapped by, their illness or CFS.

Most people, including some CFS sufferers, don't have a clear understanding or appreciation of Chronic Fatigue

Syndrome, let alone what it is like to have it. This makes any relationship between a CFS sufferer and non-sufferer a tenuous one.

To illustrate my point, last week a card came to me in the mail from my sister Mena. She had enclosed a newspaper clipping that portrayed a gripping tale of a musician who was struggling with CFS. Along with the clipping my sister included this note, "I thought you might find this interesting. It helped me understand just how debilitating CFS is." This message of understanding arrived after six long CFS-filled years, with little prior recognition from Mena that I had any illness at all.

Mena hasn't been the only person in my world who seems to ignore my CFS; most everyone I know remains ignorant about my disease, and it has taken years for my family members to even utter the words, "Chronic Fatigue," or to acknowledge in any way that I have been suffering from an illness. This absence of acknowledgment and support has greatly strained these relationships—making our inter-actions even harder than they might otherwise have been.

Fortunately, not all CFS sufferers live far away from their families, nor do they encounter such daunting barriers built up over time due to a lack of understanding. However, if you do, I write this chapter for you.

What can we do if our family members don't seem to understand or acknowledge our CFS?

If communication is strained, or you have difficulty explaining the complexity of CFS to your family, you might try an alternative approach. Instead, try sending family members copies of short excerpts from this book (or some other source) that concisely describes your illness experience. (You may want to copy the *CFS fact sheet* or contact CFIDS for CFS pamphlets; see Resources.) Or, to help loved ones "get" what CFS feels like, have them turn to CH: 7, *CFS From the Inside*.

We all want to be understood, especially by our families. We seek their compassion—deep down desiring nothing more than their understanding and support. We may also wish they could help us, but our family may not be able to lend their assistance—no matter how much we declare our CFS needs. If that is the case with you, save your precious energy for yourself; you're going to need it. Instead of seeking help outside yourself, turn your focus inward.

When your efforts to communicate go unnoticed or are misunderstood by loved ones, let go of your need for validation or confirmation from others. It's hard, I know—it can be even harder than enduring many CFS symptoms because family is so important. We will always desire our family's love, understanding, approval, and compassion. Even so, at this time you must let go of your agenda for others and concentrate on yourself. And you know what? Your family will probably come around eventually, even if it takes years. My family did.

Why can't (or won't) your family members "see" your CFS?

Families are strong units that thrive on continuity, and family members don't like to see other family members change because it upsets the family structure and dynamic. If one person changes, as a natural consequence, the entire family unit must change. Typically, families don't like change, because it seems easier not to, or it feels threatening. However, the idea that change is threatening or even bad, is just an illusion because we all change; change is the cycle of life.

When a family member develops CFS (or any other illness), s/he unwittingly upsets the family structure. All of a sudden, one person is ill, and the rest of the family is no longer sure how to act. They don't know whether to be sympathetic, extra helpful, or act as if nothing has changed. It's really quite remarkable how unnerving illness can be for people.

Even after years of being ill myself, I am still not sure how to respond to other people's illnesses. Take, for instance, my situation with my neighbor who was recently diagnosed with cancer. While she doesn't act differently around me, I still question and second-guess myself as to how to be and what to say to around her. I know if she read this, she'd say, "C'mon, Gretchen! Snap out of it! I am still the same person." But actually she has changed, so I think I need to, as well. I want to be supportive, helpful, and loving, but surprisingly I frequently question what that looks like.

Why should the illness of others have such a profound effect on us, especially those of us with illnesses of our own?

People act strangely around illness because it scares them. They don't understand it and probably think that illness requires something different from them. Many may struggle with the insane notion that if they are around ill people, maybe they'll somehow get it, even if the illness is not contagious (and CFS does not appear to be).

Have you ever noticed that if you're around a sad person for an extended period of time, you may begin to feel a bit sad yourself? This happens because we've trained ourselves to demonstrate our caring by sharing other people's feelings. This dynamic also can occur with illness. For example, healthy people may believe they will get ill simply by being around illness, or perhaps they are simply afraid of being around an ill person because they don't know how to act or think they have to act in a way that they would rather not.

Have you ever noticed that people tend to avoid being around sick people? People simply don't like illness of any kind. Chronic illness is especially disliked because it lasts a long time (or in rare cases, forever). Family members hate to experience having any member ill, especially with something as elusive as CFS. So unconsciously they reason if they don't see the CFS, it won't really be there! It's quite common for people to respond to other people's illness (and CFS) through denial. (Some people even do this with their own illness.)

Denial is something we all practice from time to time when faced with colossal challenges. It's hard being on either end of CFS, but it's worse when you get yourself wrapped up in someone else's game of denial. If those around you deny your CFS, you're better off leaving them to their ways, and concentrating on what's real for you.

Throughout my CFS journey, I frequently endured relationships seeped in denial of my illness. My family seemed unaware of my illness most of the time. My friends seemed to disappear during the hardest periods of my CFS. And even my husband, much of the time, appeared ignorant or insensitive to my CFS reality. Consequently, I too struggled to validate my CFS. Between my family and husband not "getting it," to my friends who never called, I too, began to question if CFS was really happening to me, despite mountains of evidence to the contrary.

Do not let yourself be swayed by other people's denial. It is hard enough having CFS, but it's nearly impossible to heal when you're in denial. As you deny yourself the validation you deserve, you begin to question if you're going crazy or just trying to "get out of doing things," imagining your symptoms, and making them all up. All of these destructive thoughts, though they affirm your desire to be well, only drain your energy.

To deny your illness and resume life as it was before CFS will only exacerbate your illness. To help yourself heal, it's best that you confirm that, *yes you have CFS*. Voicing the truth of your experience will empower you. You can validate yourself even when others do not.

Validation has been something I've sought consistently from my loved ones. As I cried for it, I expended a lot of my energy outward, wishing and trying to change others. It's much more powerful, productive, and healing to turn that energy inward and let go of needing specific outcomes from other people. You cannot change others, but you can change yourself. You can be the person who validates your experience.

When you have CFS, you are sick and no longer able to do what you once did, nor able to take care of things as well. Let your friends, family, and your partner know this in the best way you can, even if it means facing their denial.

If you grew up as I did, in a family characterized by independence, then even when you're ill, you will continue to take care of yourself. Maybe you are a parent, wife, or someone who has typically done a lot for other people. You may be a caretaker, someone who frequently puts others' needs before her own, and may not be used to caring for yourself; or, like me, have gotten along without assistance most of your life. As such, you're able to care for yourself and are expected to do it on your own. Now with CFS, you may be tired of taking care of everything and everyone all the time. Instead, you want to be taken care of and wonder when it will be your turn to be nurtured, instead of always being the nurturer. Now, it is your turn to be nurtured.

Because my husband is as busy as ever with work and school, and grew up in a household where he was constantly taken care of; he unfortunately has little time to help me, and knows little about how to care-take others (or himself). Consequently, I must take care of myself.

Given that self-care is essential to healing, if no one can help you care for yourself, than you must learn to do it for yourself. Self-care, whether ill or not, expresses self-appreciation, and in CFS, self-care is a necessary aspect of the healing journey.

Having CFS can mean being even more alone than before. When you cannot participate in things you once did, you obviously cannot socialize a great deal. Talking may also be difficult because of CFS' impact on the brain, especially the memory, speech portions. In Kenny, (94), Timothy explains that tests show that CFS impairs certain portions of the brain, especially those associated with memory and speech.

With CFS, it's nearly (if not entirely) impossible to commit to anything. Our bodies don't operate on set schedules—or at least not the one on which the rest of the world operates. We may sleep when others are awake; our minds may work at the darkest hours and then become immobilized in the evening when others want to interact with us or expect us to be somewhere.

Family expectations run not only from my family members to me, but in the reverse direction as well. I, too, have expectations of them. With expectations, I assure you, comes frustration and disappointment.

People rarely do what we hope, so when they do, it's best if we simply are grateful. When they don't, it's best if we can open our hearts and let go, or at least not respond with resentment. Remember: people cannot read your mind, and they certainly don't understand what you are feeling. So you must do your best to communicate your needs thus helping others to help you.

From the outset of my CFS, I expected my family to understand, acknowledge, and show compassion toward my illness and me. However, over the years their actions shattered many of the expectations I had of them. I think a part of me truly believed that by having CFS, it was finally my turn to get some attention and be cared for. I've craved this attention from my family for years, only to be reminded that this is not what they have in mind. The lesson is still painful, but it urges me to "Let go!"

When our families can't give us the love, attention, and recognition for that which we yearn, that which we seek, than it's best that we turn to those who can: be they friends, spouse, co-workers, church members, support group members, cats, dogs, our children... whomever. While it would be wonderful if the support we needed came from our family or those closest to us, when the reality indicates otherwise, reach elsewhere. Love is always available from somewhere; place your heart there and support yourself.

Gems

When your efforts to communicate go unnoticed or are misunderstood, let go of your need for validation and confirmation.

Why can't family "see" your CFS?
Family members don't like when other members change because it upsets the family structure and dynamic.

People act funny around illness because it scares them and they lack understanding.

To deny your CFS and resume life as it was before will only exacerbate your illness. To help yourself heal, confirm your CFS.

23
A PERFECT CFS COMPANION: YOUR CAT

We are human-beings not human-doings.

Neale Donald Walsch

I hope that you are as lucky as I am and have cats. Cats are the best CFS companions. I know because I cannot imagine having CFS without them. They have made the isolation of CFS more than bearable. They are perfect CFS companions because their purr reminds you of their loving presence, and the warmth of their acceptance. They accept you totally and unconditionally. They completely love you now, the same as always. Only now, your cats may love your lifestyle even more, because you are living more in-line with theirs—"catnapping" throughout the day, laying around when ordinarily you'd be out and about or busy with household or business tasks. Now, you and your felines can catnap together!

Maybe not all cats are affectionate sleeper-types like my Sage. Your cat may be more active—a prowler, or independent like my Rita. More than likely, however, your cat is aware of your change. And, your cat, unlike your human comrades, senses your need for a cozy, quiet, ever-present, always loyal, totally accepting companion. The bottom line is your cat can help you.

I am lucky because my Sage is such a cat; she sleeps beside me whenever I wish (and sometimes when I don't). She constantly reminds me that I am still wonderful, loveable, and nice to be around. In fact, my current lifestyle appeals to her restful composure, and she enjoys joining me for frequent bed rest and relaxation.

Cats don't have the human need to "do" anything rather they are the epitome of "being" creatures. They can lay around sleeping day and night, remaining perfectly at peace with themselves and the world—having nothing to do, nothing to prove. Cats are the poster children for "being-ness."

The "art of being" is a beautiful, peaceful state of feeling good without having to do anything. Meditating, relaxing, and contemplating are all ways to "be." These are well known practices that are acceptable forms of simply "being" in our society. Just lying around is not. CFS champions the idea that simply *being* is a worthwhile expression, in and of itself. CFS demands you actually stop and just *be*. Rest. Get cozy with your wonderful model of "being-ness"— your cat.

Let your cat teach you how wonderful being in bed can be. Bask in the peace; bask in the warmth of your blanket and the gentle purr of your feline friend. You need rest, so why not get cozy with the best of CFS friends (your cat), and let yourself discover a wonderful side to illness—getting in touch with what it means to *be*.

It's all very simple. You lay where you are and become absolutely aware of everything and nothing. In bed, with nothing to do but lie there, notice whatever catches your attention. If your attention is continually drawn to pain or negative thoughts, try rerouting your awareness to your cat. Your cat is nothing but ease, love, and acceptance of you, and focused on nothing more than you in this moment.

Blessed cat. Blessed *be*. Let your cat teach you how to *be* and how to accept the non-doing reality of CFS.

GEMS

Cats are the best CFS companions because they accept you and your condition totally and unconditionally.

Cats have nothing to do, nothing to prove; they are poster children for being-ness.

The "art of Being" is a beautiful, peaceful state of feeling good without having to do anything. Meditating, relaxing, and contemplating are all ways to be.

24
Separating Self From CFS

We are all born under the same sky, but we don't all have the same horizon.

Marcus Aurelius

Yesterday, when the phonology test I was taking turned out different from what I had expected and from what I had studied for, I panicked. Fear enveloped me. Today, I can't even recall my thoughts, and there were thoughts, thoughts of fear, of panic, and of fleeing. Somehow, amidst this panic, I managed to quiet my mind long enough to focus on the test and complete it. So it went: I'd pick up my pen, think a little about the question, a question I believed I knew little about, and then attempt to answer it. During each answer, fearful thoughts crept into my mind and flashes of "I can't do this!" reverberated inside me. Though I did my best, managing to complete what I considered an unfair exam, my panic paralyzed my brain at regular intervals. At those times, I found myself wondering: *Is this me or my Chronic Fatigue?*

That's the million-dollar question, isn't it? That's the question I will attempt to answer for you. The question, *Is it you or CFS?*, could be one question you're likely to ask yourself many times throughout your CFS journey. It may be a question that troubles you, as it has me. So, let's consider it.

Is what I am experiencing me or my CFS?

Many of the emotional/psychological imbalances of CFS masquerade as symptoms of depression, anxiety-related illness, and possibly other mental illnesses. What makes it so difficult to differentiate the effects of CFS on the psychological and emotional states is that these symptoms are not measurable, testable, and can be attributed to many simultaneous system failures. The brain and its many chemical reactions (involving neurotransmitters), affect our thoughts and feelings, as well as every bodily system (nervous, endocrine, circulatory, digestive, skeletal, respiratory, skin, urinary, reproductive, and muscular).

If you learn of bad news, the news is transformed from negative brain images into chemicals; these, in turn, are sent to places in your body as far away as your intestines and may create intestinal upset or some other symptom. Just as our brain impacts our bodily systems, so too the reverse is true, with our bodily systems affecting our brain. Our entire body, with all its organs and systems, is comprised of a beautifully interwoven, never-ending communication loop. We see this interweaving when nutritional deficiencies cause mental illness, for example. Specifically, some depressions may be linked to low blood sugar and some anxiety disorders (panic attacks, claustrophobia) can be attributed to allergies or poor diet. Mood disorders, such as bipolar (or manic depression), typically correlate with a serotonin (neurotransmitter in the brain) disturbance and an underlying nutritional deficiency. Null, (95).

Null, (95) explains how feelings such as lack of control, anger, and worthlessness may be rooted in hormonal imbalances, decreased serotonin levels, nutritional deficiency, hypoglycemia, diabetes, or allergies. So when your emotions grow to the extreme, and you find yourself making mountains out of molehills, there's a good chance (CFS and one of its many physical imbalances) are playing a role.

How, in the face of so many variables, do I know if my panic and inability to cope are simply my own reactions to my world or a result of my CFS and its imbalances? Do I really need to know the answer to this question? If you experience these types of feelings frequently, then, yes, you need to know; you need to know so you don't blame yourself for something that is a part of you, but is *not* you. You need to know, so you can help realign yourself physically, so that you are healthier mentally and emotionally. You need to know so you can explain to your loved ones what is transpiring, so they can be more compassionate or distant (if the situation warrants such).

In the summer of 1997, my husband Carl returned home after an eight-week intensive workshop, and he came home a changed man. I have never missed someone so profoundly as when he was absent that summer, and I have never felt so much anger toward any one person as I felt toward him when he returned.

When Carl came back, my idea of what we were had vanished and transformed. Who he was and how we were were radically transformed by his changes, and I was not ready for the "new" him or the different us. I wanted to go back in time, back to the Carl I had known (although deep down I recognized that wouldn't have sufficed either). I wanted to turn back the pages of time even if what we once had wasn't perfect. The man who now stood before me was a stranger, and that my husband could become a stranger terrified me.

What was so hard about Carl's return was how much his changes threatened me. I felt like an angry banshee, unable to control my emotions. He continually "pushed my buttons," to test his newfound growth and ability to stay "in love" amidst my reactions of anger or whatever emotion I expressed (and he even did this intentionally at times, he later admitted to me). The more Carl remained calm and distant, the more enraged I became. Carl remembers me getting angry at least ten times a day that summer. Regretfully, I would have to agree.

The interesting thing about all this rage is that it wasn't necessarily new, but it was very out of control at a time when I, too, was physically very out of balance, (yet working on my healing wholeheartedly). At the time, CFS was my main reality. So, too, were depression, feelings of worthlessness, and great confusion. I was not in a healthy state, and my emotions were greatly impacted by my physical imbalances.

Even today I am not sure whether the severity of my anger was tied to B vitamin or magnesium deficiencies, food allergies, hypoglycemia, hypothyroidism, overactive adrenal glands, or hormonal imbalances. What I do know is that as I became healthier, I also became happier and my emotions smoothed out and were less volatile.

Now, my health has improved, and when faced with extreme stress, I find I am better able to face it without falling apart. Clearly, my past out-of-control feelings, were, in part, exacerbated by my CFS.

As already indicated by my story, CFS sometimes expresses itself through chaotic emotions. Just as we cannot truly control the physical reality of CFS; to some degree we cannot control the emotional/mental impacts of it either. This is not to say that I encourage feelings of victimization or lack of personal responsibility. Instead, I am merely attempting to illustrate the complex picture of Chronic Fatigue Syndrome and help you understand what is yours, and what isn't.

At some point in your illness journey, it will prove helpful to know that your emotional extremes are not *you* and not *your fault*. This absolution will lift a burden, one which may be too heavy, and not entirely yours to carry.

When chaotic feelings do arise: do what you can to identify your imbalances; do what you can to heal. When you are caught inside an emotional roller coaster, try to give yourself what few others will: acceptance, love, and support. You can embrace yourself and know that you are doing the best you can. Try to understand the chaos, or at least accept it for now.

Sometimes, CFS is so pervasive throughout your being that you cannot respond as you used to or would like to; that is the reality for now. As you experience better health, your state of mind and emotions will smooth out. Trust the process and inform loved ones of your emotional fragility. As you begin to heal imbalances, your emotions will settle down and fall in-line.

Know what is you, and what is CFS, and know that you are not dramatizing when you have extreme reactions to your imbalances because from "where you sit" things feel pretty crazy. Take heart, over time you will feel more in-balance.

GEMS

Just as we cannot really control the physical reality of CFS; we also cannot always control the emotional/mental impacts of it.

Know what is you and what is CFS. Know that you are not dramatizing, but rather reacting to the imbalances that are beyond your control.

25
DECIDING TO HEAL

What lies behind us, and what lies before us, are tiny matters compared to what lies within us.

Ralph Waldo Emerson

It's really very simple: you can decide that you want to be ill and a victim of your unfortunate, unfair circumstances, or you can decide you want to heal and take charge of your illness. Taking charge in no way means that you alone are responsible for your recovery (as there may be larger forces at work that ultimately decide the "when and how" you heal). However, it does mean that you are ready to heal and are taking action toward your healing.

This past spring when my Mom came to visit, she told me a story about a woman with CFS that illustrates some of our power in the matter of our healing.

One day, my Mom, Judy, had gone into town to work when she ran into Sue. Over the years, Mom and Sue had shared several conversations about Sue's CFS, as well as my own. Typically, Sue would share with my Mom the despair she felt, as well as her feelings of isolation; hers was a story filled with hopelessness. "No one," Sue bemoaned, "No one understands."

Judy would listen, and update Sue on my progress with CFS, usually an equally sad story. And that is how it would go—their sharing and bond founded on CFS blues.

One day the following spring, however, when Judy bumped into Sue, the usual chain of events was broken. When Sue asked my Mom how I was doing, Judy enthusiastically replied, "Gretchen has really improved!" Instantly, acting as if Judy had uttered the unspeakable, the bond was severed and Sue backed away. Unable to hide her disappointment, Sue chose to hide herself instead. Once again, Sue was alone in her suffering because my Mom no longer shared in Sue's vision of CFS as "that ugly, awful disease from whence there is no return." Instead, Judy saw that people do improve and recover from CFS as she witnessed her own daughter working with her illness rather than against it.

In Sue's case, the notion of CFS being anything but bleak was beyond her imagination because she had learned to thoroughly identify herself with CFS, with an illness that was all negative. In Sue's mind, she had no control over her situation and gloom, and this mindset prevented her from seeing another person's empowerment as cause for celebration. Sue, in some very real way, wanted to remain "stuck" in seeing herself as a powerless victim of a dreadful disease. Author Caroline Myss calls this attitude, *nursing our wounds*, and Sue epitomized a person doing just that.

Most CFSers begin their CFS journey as a "Sue," someone who feels and acts like a victim. I too periodically fall back into the victim mindset myself, feeling that, "My entire being has been taken over by a fatigue which I can do nothing about!"

Fortunately, I can only stomach being in the darkness for so long. Eventually, I decide to step into the light and take charge of changing my reality. There exists little that is more powerful than our will to decide: we decide what we think, what we say, and more importantly, how we'll act. To change my CFS experience all I had to do was *decide to heal.*

Deciding to heal is the act of making up your mind that you want to get better. Next, it's making the decision that you can indeed get better. Third, it's taking any and all actions that you believe will lead to your recovery.

Healing is as much an internal, mental, and spiritual process as it is a physiological body experience. When you convert from victim to victor, you have mobilized not only your spirit, but also the very cells in your body. It is impossible to affect only one part of our beings; when we think, feel, speak, or act, we trigger reactions within our minds, bodies, and souls. Our multi-faceted selves are so interconnected that changing thoughts and attitudes in turn changes our physical body.

I decided to heal after enduring two difficult, unhappy, lonely years of suffering. My worst year, when I was truly at my sickest, was the year I lived in Quebec. As bad as my illness was, my mindset was worse. I was convinced that Quebec was "out to get me." It seemed every time I attempted to do something—whether it was go to the grocery store, the mechanic, or to the big city of Montreal—I was in for a challenge. While at the grocery store, I'd lose my way in the parking lot and forget where I had parked. At the mechanics, they would discover two more things wrong with our van, and that would raise the bill and deteriorate my mood. Driving to Montreal, I'd miss my exit, get stuck in traffic, and drive around, panicked, exhausted, and hungry.

Nothing came easy. Oh, how I hated living there! If all of the above weren't bad enough, factor in the language ordeal and brutal weather. I hated Quebec, and that of course only seemed to make Quebec "hate" me in return. My life while in Quebec was a year filled with suffering.

After that bleak, difficult year, I decided I was done with misery and struggle and was ready to be happy and well. When we moved to Colorado, I brought a changed attitude. The move, no doubt, helped me to help myself, but ultimately, I had decided it was time. One only has to go through so much darkness before the light finds its way in.

Deciding to heal is as easy or difficult as we make it. Even when our health eludes us with persistent imbalances and symptoms, we can take control of our minds and beliefs. If the reality you're experiencing doesn't support your healthy thoughts, look elsewhere to help reinforce the vision you wish to create. If you feel ready to heal and there are no fears holding you back, this is a good time to resource others who think positively. Talk to people about how you are healing and about how you want to heal. Surround yourself with people who are supportive of your getting better. If you have been relating to people from a place of "poor, pitiful me" and getting sympathy for your demise, realize this kind of "support" is no longer beneficial. To quote Caroline Myss, *you are nursing wounds*, not healing them. Surround yourself instead with empathetic people who will encourage your progress in healing, not promote feelings of disempowerment.

Deciding to heal begins after you've embraced your illness and accepted it into your life. Once you accept your illness, you are now empowered to decide that you no longer see yourself as needing illness in your life. You believe you can get better and are ready to get better. Part of getting better and deciding to heal includes trust and allowance.

When your body persists in having illness and symptoms, part of your response can be to trust the temporary "down" days that appear like setbacks or relapses, but are simply another cycle in your healing process. (For more on how to cope at these times, read CH: 13, *Surviving the CFS Lows*)

Know too that everything cycles. Everyone, healthy or ill passes through times of movement (change) and stagnation (static states). An integral aspect to any journey is a curvy, bumpy road filled with light, interspersed by darkness. Each time we move through our darkness, having gained new perspectives or insights, we attract more light into our lives.

We must learn to trust the process, while maintaining our determination to heal. We then open ourselves up, allowing for times when our body is severely ill, knowing that being ill today does not mean being ill tomorrow. In fact, being ill today may actually mean we're freeing ourselves from our illness. The mere fact that we experience symptoms is evidence that our bodies are working and fighting the unwanted. When a virus overtakes us, for example, our bodies' immune systems respond through feverish fires. These fires burn the virus out of us. Thus, the fever (symptom) is not the enemy, but rather our friend. Keep this in mind when you feel overpowered by symptoms.

When our bodies call for our attention and care, our most healing response is to allow our bodies exactly what they crave—full attention and loving-kindness.

Most of us have at some time neglected to allow for "down" days or hours and have found ourselves in relapse. I prefer to say your body is just in need of rest. If you have made progress and suddenly are "stopped" by a day or week of "down time," try using this as a time to thank your body for all the healing it has done thus far. Trust that this week of slow symptom-filled days is simply your body's way of regaining equilibrium after having made so much progress! One cannot keep moving up a mountain without ever taking a rest. Your body needs a break; breaks are natural stages in any healing cycle.

All CFS journeys alternate between periods of healing (traversing the mountains), with periods of resting, (nesting in the valley of symptoms). Trust the waves; allow for the peaks and valleys. Keep on climbing, and remember to allow for breaks along the way. When you have decided it's time to heal, that very decision will mobilize you and help you on your healing journey.

GEMS

It is very simple: you can decide that you want to be ill and a victim of your unfortunate, unfair circumstances, or you can decide you want to heal and take charge of your illness.

Deciding to heal is the act of making up your mind that you want to get better.

There exists little that is more powerful than our will to decide. We decide what we want to think; we decide what we say, and most important, we decide how we'll act.

Deciding to heal is as easy or difficult as we make it. Even when our health eludes us with persistent imbalances and symptoms, we can take control of our minds and beliefs. If the reality you are experiencing doesn't support your healthy thoughts, look elsewhere to help reinforce the reality you wish to create.

26
NOURISH THY SOUL

If we are not doing the job or leading the life we enjoy, our mind is constantly holding the thought, "I wish I weren't here." As our body is a slave to our mind, our body will then start getting us out of whatever we want to get out of. The first step is illness.

Andrew Mathews

In today's world, health is an important facet of our lives. When we think of health, we usually think of just our bodies such as our dietary choices and exercise, but health also includes spiritual nourishment. In fact, weekends are society's way of bringing about nourishment of our soul. For example, weekends filled with fun, enjoying ourselves and having the freedom to do what we want, when we want, nourishes the soul. We all seek a life that includes some kind of soul nourishment even if most of us are calling it by another name, "fun."

For me, fun means: relaxation, freedom, no commitment, and most of all, having fun means being able to play and experience joy. "Having fun" encompasses all forms of activity and is probably more about a state of mind than any specific activity. The problem is we all associate certain activities with fun, or by contrast, with toil. When in fact any action can we be fun if we think it so.

What does fun have to do with Chronic Fatigue Syndrome, you may be asking? My answer is, *a lot. Fun* is one form of nourishment—soul nourishment—that is essential to health and well-being.

More than likely, soul nourishment was something understated in your life before CFS. Really busy, driven people tend to find less time for fun due to the over-emphasis they place on work and/or responsibilities. The same people may even forget entirely about nurturing themselves. "Having fun" is not about work, accomplishment, or having to *be* anything or anyone at any particular time, despite the importance of these roles in our lives.

Soul nourishment is a funny thing. Interestingly enough, our society both glorifies and abhors the idea of taking care of our souls. We go out of our way to emphasize the importance of work, accomplishment, and titles, admiring people who drive themselves, doing a myriad of things, and appearing to have it all. Yet, we rarely admire the man who chooses to take a low-paying, part-time job to allow himself more time to increase relaxation or family-time. Even while idolizing "successful" people, we simultaneously crave and glorify "fun." Notice how our favorite days of the week tend not to be Mondays. "Thank God it's Friday!" we say, and mean it. All of us love weekends because it's our time to do what we want (mostly). Or, it's a time to "catch up" at home on things we haven't had time to do during the week.

If you look at our advertising, rarely does it glorify the workplace. Instead, it portrays "the good life" as laughing with friends, sitting at a bar, enjoying nature, traveling to intriguing places, drinking, relaxing...you know—"having a good time." Rarely do we associate our good times with being at work. Instead, we look forward to our weekends and vacations with great anticipation and excitement. We celebrate them. In other words, we nourish ourselves on the weekends/holidays in ways that feel good. That's what nourishment is—doing things that foster our "feeling good," and nourishes our soul.

It's sad that in today's world, we have created our lives in such a way that we emphasize the importance of work while simultaneously desiring fun and dichotomizing the two. If, on the other hand, we were enjoying ourselves at work, we wouldn't have created such a dichotomy between work and "free" time—between getting things done and having fun.

We believe, unfortunately, that we need to be stressed and serious in order to "get it done," thereby structuring our lives in such a way that work is toil, while "time off" is pleasurable and relaxing. It's a crazy, convoluted way of life, yet it's so pervasive that we never stop to question the insanity of it all.

What's insane is the perception that work has to be a struggle; work is not enjoyable and, in order to get things done, we must suffer. With such a perception/reality, it's no wonder we desire the times when we don't "have to work," time when we can "let our hair down," wear the clothes we love, and do the things we enjoy. We all need these times, because pleasure creates happiness, and happiness is what life is all about. God didn't create a world full of creatures so they could simply suffer; no way. Rather, joy is intrinsic to our nature and can come from the things we give to ourselves when we are at work *and* when we are at play.

Our nature is not to be unhappy, struggling, stressed-out individuals. We have simply created this experience for ourselves because of what we believe we *should* do or who we *should* be in our lives. Our beliefs about work are ours to change if we choose.

In contrast to the current extreme work ethic, our nature is to be less stressed and our souls yearn to return to that nature. Unfortunately, we have created lives that are stressful, having created a world in which we feel "we have to work," but would rather be "playing." Many of us work at jobs we hate, seeing no alternative. We're trapped, or so we think. And as we believe, so we live.

Alternatives don't just happen. We must believe in them and work to create them. We are powerful creators and we either choose how we live, or we limit ourselves by choosing not to decide. Either way, how we live is ultimately our choice.

Stress is a huge contributor to our ill health and our unhappiness. Stress is self-imposed, self-created, and optional. (I realize that this last assertion is controversial and there are many things in life that we do not choose. However, in any given situation, no matter how bad, there always exist several options open to us, and that permits us to choose our stress level.)

Life was not meant to be so stressful. Human beings have created immense stress. How many wild animals experience stress like we do? How much stress do you suppose humans have created? The bottom line is we created our stress. Now, it's up to us to "un-create" it by putting a stop to it in our lives.

To be healthy, we need to change, change our perceptions about work and play, and change our actions. We need to nourish our souls as much as we do our bodies and our minds. Nourishing the soul takes as many forms as nourishing the body. Look around the world at the different cultures and how each approaches the food they eat. There are countless healthy diets, each different according to culture and local agriculture. The same is true about how you can "feed" your soul. What matters most is not *how*, but *if*.

Anyone who makes her work her passion, is nourishing herself. (I am a strong advocate for doing this, and I believe that each of us was put on earth to follow our passions.) If it seems impossible to do what you love for work, than at least love what you do the rest of the time. If even doing that seems impossible, than change how you perceive the notion of "doing what you love" and learn to love doing anything. Enjoyment is a state of mind. Enjoyment comes from what you think about what you're doing, as much as from the activity itself.

We are meant to enjoy our lives. That enjoyment nourishes us. Nourishment in all forms is essential to our being. We need soul nourishment as much as physical nourishment. To nourish yourself, do what you love or love what you do, and learn to be relaxed and present in whatever space or place you find yourself. Embrace yourself and embrace the moment. Joy and nourishment for your soul is not anywhere else but here.

You can nourish yourself right now by deciding to love where you are right now. Loving or embracing is not dependent upon certain conditions; it's dependent upon your decision to love. Decide to relax. Decide to do what you want. Decide to enjoy where you are, even if it's being severely ill with Chronic Fatigue Syndrome.

Let go of the "have-tos" and the "shoulds," and embrace who you are and where you are now. Enjoy the amazing, miraculous creation of life and the nature around you; and realize that even if you can't get out of bed right now, you can decide that's fine. When all is fine; when you embrace yourself and your circumstance; you nourish your soul, and in so doing, you nourish your body.

GEMS

Fun is one form of soul nourishment and is essential to health and well-being. Having fun is not about work, accomplishment, or having to be any one or thing.

We have created a polarized world where we glorify work while simultaneously desiring fun and "free" time. In our minds, we believe we cannot have work and fun at the same time. In order to get things done we must suffer.

Stress is a huge contributor to our ill health and unhappiness. It is self-imposed, self-created, and optional.

To nourish your soul, do what you love or love what you do, and learn to relax and be present wherever you find yourself.

27
NOURISH THY BODY

The most frequently purchased foods, comprising the most popular American meal, are hamburgers, french-fries, a small salad, coffee, and soft drinks. The nutritional content of such a meal is questionable. However, the consumption of foods that are even less nutritious than these, such as "snack foods" and "junk foods" is even more a concern from the nutritional point of view.

Rudolph Ballentine

When I reflect on my CFS healing journey and ask myself what has been most healing, two key components come to mind: 1) changing my diet, and 2) altering my beliefs [though there have been many contributing factors to my healing including: 1) allowing myself to *be*, 2) healing a hormonal imbalance through both hormones and acupuncture, 3) healing hypothyroidism through natural hormones then tyrosine/kelp, 4) healing a magnesium and B-vitamin deficiency through supplementation, and 5) healing a sleep disturbance through magnesium, Chinese medicine, 5-HTP, and light therapy.]

The Importance of Diet

If you eat typical American fare, changing your diet is essential to your healing (please see the movie *Supersize*

Me). When first faced with needing to change my diet, I was reluctant because I didn't fully grasp the significance food intake bears on CFS. Nor, did I want to give up foods that gave me pleasure. Also, I thought (but now realize otherwise) that what I ate was relatively healthy. Compared to most Americans, that was true. I didn't eat much in the way of fried foods, junk foods, and I never ate red meat. I rarely drank soda and savored only one or two cups of coffee a day. In spite of all that, I did typically start my day with an unhealthy dose of sugar, fat, and caffeine, and never stopped to think about what I was ingesting. My standard breakfast consisted of coffee or a latte, juice, and a muffin or scone.

Now, I realize how little this meal truly offered in the way of nutrients. I see that my former breakfasts were laden with sugar, fat, and caffeine. And like many people in our society who want to rationalize certain dietary choices, I tried to convince myself that coffee was good for me. (And there is research to bear this popular misconception out. In fact, almost whatever diet you choose, you can find research to support it.)

Contrary to hopes, neither sugar nor caffeine provide nutrients. Instead, they provide empty, short-lived "pseudo-energy." The energy we feel after consuming sugar and caffeine stems from the initial surge of insulin and adrenaline they cause, but these later plummet.

Sugar provides a rush of energy as soon as you eat it, but shortly thereafter you crash into a sugar low caused by feeding your body simple sugars that are digested immediately and not utilized efficiently by the body. After the initial rush of energy sugar consumption causes, your energy level will drop, and your body will still crave nutrients.

To help you mask this sugar-produced "crash," you may rush to the nearest café for a caffeine fix. This choice will temporarily raise your adrenaline levels, and due to coffee's diuretic nature, will flush your system of the important vitamins: B's and C, and the minerals: calcium, potassium, magnesium, sodium, iron, and zinc. Edwards (92). The bad thing about this combination is not only are you consuming substances lacking essential nutrients, but there's the added insult of consuming substances that rob you of nutrients already in your body. Caffeine and sugar do both.

It is not easy to question our diets, because we are surrounded by masses eating the same or worse. Fortunately, we, individuals can make our own choices, and more and more people are making conscious efforts to shift eating patterns. So, the first step here is to ask yourself: *Is my diet healthy?* Then, *Do I eat a well-balanced diet with several meals a day comprised of fresh fruits, vegetables, whole grains, healthy fats and proteins? Do I experience regular intestinal upset in the form of bloating, gas, pain, and constipation? Do I have regular bowel movements at least once a day? Do I feel better or worse after I eat?* Your answers to these questions may help you identify if your diet is truly healthy.

What we eat is incredibly important, equally important

are the manner in which we eat and our thoughts and emotions surrounding our eating. First, let's consider more closely *what* we eat.

In 1996, when my doctor suggested I go on an "elimination diet"* and take supplements, I had no trouble taking the supplements. I did, however, wonder how eating a very limited, highly restrictive diet would help me. Not only did the diet feel like an insurmountable task, but it also meant giving up all my favorite foods.

Today, it's hard for me to fathom how I could not have understood the importance of diet to health, but years ago I simply was not ready to "get it." At the time, I had already lost so much, and changing my diet just seemed like another loss—not a potential source of healing.

So, what is there to 'get?' Do you have to go on an elimination diet, too? First, you need to understand how your body needs micro and macronutrients to function. All bodily functions, chemical reactions, and mental processes require that we take in nutrients that facilitate their performance. We also need fuel in the form of energy to give us vitality. Nutrients and calories obtained from our food, work to keep us alive and help us to thrive. Just as a car doesn't run without gas and a plant doesn't grow without light, we don't live without nutrients and fuel in the form of healthy food.

A healthy diet is important to everyone, yet somehow many people manage to function on questionable,

---

* Elimination Diets: These diets are intended for people with food allergies or sensitivities; they help uncover specific allergens and allow the body to heal from their impact.

unhealthy fare. *Why can't you and I get away with eating the way others do—have our cake and eat it, too, so to speak?* People with CFS are different. Our CFS bodies are already working hard to rebalance our weakened systems. Our immune, nervous, and digestive systems are not what they could be, nor what they used to be. To aid these systems in their work, and to help ourselves receive the corresponding emotional improvement, we need to feed ourselves well.

I don't recommend starting with a complete elimination diet if it feels overwhelming. But, I can now affirm through my own healing, the benefits of going through such a program and making dietary changes.

Many of us suffer from digestive-related disorders. We experience excess gas, bloating, constipation, and/or diarrhea. These digestive symptoms are not a natural part of living; they indicate digestive problems, be they dietary, nutritional, allergic, or parasitic in nature. Often, such symptoms are the result of a fiber-less, nutrient-deficient diet, typical of the American way of eating. They may be a result of a deficiency in digestive enzymes (which are obtained through raw fruits and vegetables), or due to food allergies/sensitivities.

I discovered that I suffered from all of the above, (except parasites), and that going on an elimination diet, and later a yeast-free diet, helped me to identify my specific allergens and uncover a yeast infection. Also, by eliminating alcohol, sugar, and coffee from my diet, my overall health and emotions improved.

When I first tried the Candida diet, (eliminating all sugars, dairy, wheat products, and any fermented foods), I was amazed, when after a week into it, I suffered a day of what nutritionists call "yeast die-off." I literally felt like I was suffering from withdrawal. All I could think about, all I wanted was something, anything with sugar in it. I was irritable, distraught, and unable to focus; I felt as if I'd gone totally insane!

On that day, I discovered how much my body relied on, and was, in fact, addicted to sugar. That experience was enough to convince me that I was doing the right thing. I then decided that if sugar had that kind of hold on me, it was not meant to be part of my healing journey. I soon felt the benefits of clearing my system of its overgrowth of yeast caused by an overly sugary diet, lacking in nutrients and friendly flora, and my energy and digestion soon improved.

That was not the only strict diet I tried. Others followed, some more rigid and more difficult; and yet after each one, I noticed that my energy always increased. Admittedly, when I first encountered these diets, I cringed, but my will to follow them grew with each added day of better health and increased energy. Eventually, I would give up every vice/food addiction I had ever had, namely coffee and sugar, as well as wheat and dairy. (Eventually I brought all of these back into my diet in moderation.)

How Digestion works and why it is important

What you eat starts to break down in the mouth long before reaching the intestines, and causes chemical reactions—good and bad—depending on what is consumed and how well your digestive system can extract and eliminate waste.

Our CFS Bodies, overwhelmed by digestive disturbances, cannot depend on our livers and intestines to do an adequate job of ridding our systems of unwanted chemicals (pesticides, artificial colorings, thickeners, preservatives and the like) from unhealthy diets. Instead, we need to give our bodies food rich in nutrients and low in toxins.

As it is, we already absorb enough toxins through our environment via the air we breathe, through the pesticide-laced soil in which our produce is grown, from the industrial chemicals running into our water, through our common household products and building materials, and finally via the farm animals we eat that are poisoned by antibiotics and growth hormones. Our current state of the environment urges us to pay attention; pay attention to what we eat and how our choices exacerbate or decrease stress on the planet and ourselves.

How You Eat

Not only is what we eat key, but how we eat is equally significant. Many people eat "on the run," unconsciously shoving food in their mouths and down their throats, as if they can't eat it quickly enough. Eating too fast can result in severe digestive upsets, because one may swallow excess air, resulting in unwanted gases, and the digestive enzymes in our mouths may have little chance to begin the process of breaking the food down.

As we chew, we begin the food breakdown process, because the more we chew, the more enzymes are secreted and the better the nutrients in food can be absorbed. If under-chewed food passes through our esophagus into our stomach, our stomach can become overburdened and pass the food on to the intestines, where many digestive symptoms may result such as gas, bloating, and pain. These are just some of the things that can go wrong if we eat too fast and fail to chew adequately.

Thinking about Eating

How we think about our food also influences what we eat. Eating without thinking about our food can lead us to choose easy foods, such as junk or fast foods, high in fat, sugar, salt, as well as chemicals and unnatural additives. Have you ever asked yourself why they're called "junk foods?" These foods are characteristically high in sugar, salt, fat, and chemicals in the form of coloring, flavor additives, preservatives, and thickeners. Together these ingredients make junk foods more appealing, palatable, and lead to a longer shelf life. These additives are completely unnecessary and unhealthy. Each time we ingest them, we introduce more "non-foods" into our systems that require processing and elimination, thus adding greater stress on our already-stressed digestive systems.

Giving Attention to the Meal

Not only does what we eat matter, but how we feel about our food affects our digestion of it. If you come to the table stressed, the energy needed for digestion is already spent stressing. Our bodies cannot do everything at once. If the immune system and heart are on alert, the digestive system is put on hold, thereby making eating incompatible with stress. Relaxing and taking time out to enjoy your food is as important to your health as *what* you eat.

Making meals requires attention, choice, and effort. It is not always easy, but the process of turning a meal into a ritual brings rewards. When we create a meal, we get to decide what we eat, how much we eat, and how we eat. We have the freedom to choose healthy or unhealthy foods. When we choose healthy foods, we not only do a good thing for our body; we also do a good thing for our mind and the planet.

When we create our own meals, we enjoy the added bonus of choosing products consciously. We can select products from companies we believe in. Eating consciously spawns many rewards adding pleasure to an otherwise ordinary daily activity. Eating a meal, for example can become a soulful ritual whether experienced alone or in the company of others. The whole act of selecting, preparing, and eating a meal when done deliberately with care can become nourishment for the body and soul.

I have always preferred a sit-down, slow meal to a hurried one. I enjoy sharing in conversation with others at mealtimes or sitting alone with good food before me. Meals are a very important part of my day—too important to skip, skimp on, or sail through.

I highly recommend that you learn to value a meal. Your body and soul will thank you for it.

GEMS

The first step in nourishing the body is to ask your - self: Is my diet healthy?

Why can't we have our cake and eat it too? People with CFS have bodies that are working extremely hard to rebalance. Your immune, nerv - ous and digestive systems are not what they could be, or what they used to be.

Our CFS bodies, overwhelmed by digestive dis - turbances, cannot depend on our intestines and livers to do an adequate job of ridding our systems of unwanted chemicals (pesticides, artificial colorings, thickeners, and preservatives...). Instead, we need to give our bodies food rich in nutrients and low in toxins.

Many people eat on the run, unconsciously shoving food down their throats, almost as if they can't eat quickly enough. Eating too fast can result in severe digestive upsets.

How we think about our food influences what we eat. Eating without thinking about our food choices can lead us to choose easy foods such as junk or fast food. These are loaded with fat, sugar, salt, chemicals, and unnatural additives.

Our emotional state can affect our digestion. If you enter a meal stressed, the energy needed for digestion is being used to stress. Relaxing and taking time out to enjoy your food is as important as what you eat.

28
CFS REMEDIES

Throughout my healing journey I have suffered countless symptoms. Sometimes they were so numerous, I would forget them when asked about my health. Having so many symptoms has confounded my healing process and complicated my healing. Often times when I have seen a doctor/healer, I haven't known where to begin, so I drudge up my symptoms as best as I recall in the moment. This is very stressful. Soon the stress causes memory lapse and I leave disappointed and less informed than I had hoped.

I cannot tell you how many symptom lists I have written over these past ten years, and how many ways I have diagrammed my health picture. While frustrating to no end, these symptoms have led me to better understand my body, how to heal, and ultimately to become my own empowered healer.

This is where you come in. Because CFS is complex and often overwhelming, each CFSer must take it upon him or herself to be proactive. You must go to your healer prepared, armed with symptom lists, questions, and concerns—even if that means risking your doctor labeling you a hypochondriac. (If they are that insensitive, they probably aren't the best healers.)

Your healing is up to you. That is why I have included a remedy list here, hoping to assist you—by my example—in creating your own list. Perhaps this will help you see the interconnections between symptoms and imbalances and help you realize the vast array of healing options open to you, as well as inspire you to take charge of your healing whenever possible.

To follow is a list highlighting many of the symptoms I have grappled with throughout CFS. I have included first, a list in bold of symptoms/conditions, followed by their common causes, and the treatments that most helped me or that were recommended by healing practitioners.

What has worked for me may not work for you. Know that these treatments were recommended to me by healers or were based on my own research or course-work. For this section (and throughout this book), I have consulted with local medical professionals for accuracy. Please use this list only as a guideline; consider consulting with a medical professional before trying a remedy.

FATIGUE

CFS, Candida, allergies, hypothyroidism, hyperthyroidism, anemia, weak adrenals, fibromyalgia, lupus, B12 deficiency, stress, hypoglycemia and sleep disturbances (this is not a complete list)

Possible Remedies

- Improve thyroid (thyroid hormones, iodine supplementation, tyrosine supplementation, Chinese herbs)

- Decrease/eliminate sugar, caffeine, alcohol
- Myer's cocktail (intravenous vitamin B mix administered by doctor)
- Light Therapy using blue light (especially for sleep disturbances)
- B12 shots
- Attunement
- Acupuncture
- Meditation/Visualization
- Yoga
- Walking
- Engage in energy-inducing companionship (some relationships are energy-draining)
- Watch inspiring show or movie
- Rest or get deep sleep
- Food, especially protein, veggies, complex-carbs (when it's due to hypoglycemia)
- Do anything soul inspiring

SLEEP DISTURBANCE

Brain-wave disturbances caused by hypothalamus, fibromyalgia, low blood sugar, irregular heartbeat, sinus and congestion. Verrillo, (97). Yin deficiency (Chinese medicine), circadian rhythm imbalance due to S.A.D (Seasonal Affective Disorder).

Possible Remedies

- 5-HTP
- Myer's cocktail

- Tryptophan
- Valerian
- Melatonin, use with caution because it is a hormone and its impact on the pineal gland is not greatly understood
- Take magnesium at night (also very good for cramping, nervousness, and pain)
- Over-the-counter pill "Sleep Ease," helps, but may also cause extreme drug-like state
- Ensure room is dark when you sleep
- Unwind before bed with relaxing activities that are not too loud, bright, or stimulating: read, meditate, journal, and engage in mellow conversation)

DIFFICULTY CONCENTRATING

Candida, allergies, weak adrenals, fibromyalgia, hyperthyroid, hypoglycemia, brain malfunction, and sleep deprivation.

Possible Remedies

- Good food (especially protein when it's due to hypoglycemia)
- Good deep sleep including all sleep stages
- Exercise, more oxygen gets to the brain
- Acupuncture
- Address candida, fibromyalgia, poor sleep, and stress

HEADACHES

Candida, allergies, fibromyalgia, poor sleep, stress

Possible Remedies

- Apply intense pressure on pressure point between the thumb and index finger for several minutes
- Massage high quality, organic lavender oil on head, especially where it hurts
- Diet: eat well (especially for hypoglycemia)
- Diet: what you ate could cause a headache; if chronic, you may want to keep a diet journal and note when headaches occur. They could indicate a food allergy.
- Relaxation activities
- Attunement, especially on head
- Get good sleep
- Address candida, allergies, fibromyalgia, and hypothyroidism

MEMORY

Candida, allergies, fibromyalgia, hypothyroidism

Possible Remedies

- Good sleep
- Improve thyroid (if hypothyroid, get treatment)
- Address candida, allergies, and fibromyalgia
- Acupuncture

DIZZINESS

Hypothyroidism, hypoglycemia, inner ear problem (viral), eye problems

Possible Remedies
- Good deep sleep with all stages
- Treat hypoglycemia
- Eat regular, healthy meals
- Improve thyroid if hypothyroid
- Get eyes checked
- Get inner ear checked

MOODINESS, ANXIETY

Hormonal imbalance, weak adrenals, hypoglycemia, Candida

Possible Remedies
- Decrease sugar
- Decrease, eliminate caffeine
- Good Diet: fresh veggies, fruits, whole grains, legumes, nuts/seeds
- Treat hormonal imbalance
- Exercise
- Address weak adrenals, hypoglycemia, Candida

DEPRESSION

Can be due to the losses and changes attributed to CFS, neurotransmitter deficiency, stress, lack of "soul" in life, hypoglycemia, Candida, allergies, hypothyroidism

Possible Remedies
- 5-HTP at night (amazingly effective for me)
- Saint John's Wort
- Anti-depressant

- Peppermint aromatherapy, use only high-grade, pure oils
- Address losses, changes in life
- Address meaning in life
- Deal with isolation
- Spirituality (for me *Conversations with God* books were extremely helpful)
- Creative pursuits
- Soul-inspiring activities

HYPERSENSITIVITY to light (photophobia), noise, odors

Weakened nervous system, weak adrenals, allergies, Candida

Possible Remedies

- Strengthen adrenals
- Good sleep
- For light sensitivity: wear sunglasses, avoid facing contrasting light
- Reduce stress and add relaxation activities (meditation, walking, yoga, journaling, have conversations with God)

PMS

Hormonal imbalance, poor diet, nutritional deficiencies, stress

Possible Remedies

- Treat hormonal imbalance
- Evening primrose oil capsules daily (for hormones)

- Decrease or eliminate sugar, caffeine, refined carbohydrates, junk foods, and eat organic (to avoid pesticides and hormones)
- Magnesium, good for nervous system and ability to handle stress (check blood levels)
- Exercise

CONSTIPATION

Candida, hypothyroidism, hyperthyroidism, stress

Possible Remedies

- Address thyroid
- Increase magnesium
- Address excess yeast through yeast-free diet (Candida)
- Increase fiber in diet and/or supplement with fiber
- Olive oil and lemon juice by spoonful (a few teaspoons)
- Get good sleep
- Exercise
- Breathe deeply
- Relaxation
- Reduce stress
- Personal exploration: *Is there something going on in your life that feels overwhelming, confining, or restrictive? Are you able to openly communicate your feelings? Are you allowing yourself what you need?*

ACID REFLUX

Diet, hypothyroidism, stress, eating while upset, too much HCL (hydrochloric acid) in multi-vitamin

Possible Remedies

- Eliminate acid-producing foods for a period of time: tomato-based, spicy foods, citrus, coffee
- Eat plain, organic yogurt
- Improve thyroid, if hypothyroid
- Eat slowly and peacefully

BLOATING

Hormonal imbalance, allergies, Candida, constipation

Possible Remedies

- Treat hormonal imbalance
- Magnesium
- Evening primrose oil (take capsules daily)
- Address yeast
- Address PMS
- Exercise
- Massage the large intestine (entire abdomen especially across belly just below navel)
- Yoga, only positions that are comfortable

YEAST OVERGROWTH (Candida Albicans)

Poor diet (excessive sugar and refined carbohydrates), excess alcohol, excessive antibiotic exposure

Possible Remedies

- Yeast-free diet: no sugars, caffeine, fermented foods

- Take acidophilus and bifidus daily
- Caprylic acid
- Eat fiber or take fiber supplement
- Take Swedish bitters
- Get anti-yeast prescription (Diflucan, for example)

HYPOGLYCEMIA

Poor diet, excessive sugar and refined carbohydrates

Possible Remedies

- Decrease or eliminate sugar, caffeine
- Chromium Picolinate daily
- Eat frequent small healthy snacks with non-animal proteins
- L-Glutamine

OVERHEATING

Female hormones, Chinese medicine: chi stagnation, or yin deficiency, weak adrenals

Possible Remedies

- Address hormone imbalance
- Acupuncture and Chinese herbs
- Black Cohosh
- Eat aromatic herbs (to move chi)

COLD FEET

Poor circulation, hypothyroidism

Possible Remedies

- Address thyroid

- Baths
- Foot baths
- Hot tub
- Foot massage
- Exercise
- Cayenne pepper, stimulates circulation

29
CUTTING DOWN THE CFS TREE:
FROM CFS TO HEALTH

Our present perceptions are so colored by the past that we are unable to see the immediate happenings in our lives without distortions and limitations. With willingness, however, we can reexamine who we think we are in order to achieve a new and deeper sense of real identity.

Gerald Jampolsky

You know that you have reached a crossroads when you have physically reached the time of *reemergence*, a time when you have mostly healed your CFS. Now you emerge from your past life of fatigue and hibernation to revisit the world of society, of *doing*. You find yourself beginning to take on more and more activities, responsibility, and commitment. As you do, you discover that part of you still lives in the CFS mindset. Old thoughts and beliefs created from a physically compromised place continue to exert themselves in your mind, giving way to questions and uncertainty. The questions sound something like, *"What am I capable of? Which of my feelings and thoughts are real and based on the current truth? Which ones are remnants from years with fatigue and all that came from that lifestyle?"*

I have now entered the *reemergence* phase. I find myself walking across the Colorado State University campus, remembering when such a walk was a monumental task. I dash up the three flights of stairs to the third floor where the English Department lives, catching my breath and recalling a time when being inside a school building meant navigating labyrinths of unending generic doors, a task that quickly led to anxiety, sometimes panic.

Now, I am a student back in the familiar arena of education, but thrown into new territory, a CFS crossroads. Like the illness that keeps each of us inside a lonely world, this place of transition can be equally lonely.

As I try to reclaim a life that I feel ready for, I encounter frequent thoughts that stem from my CFS experience— thoughts that once made sense given CFS; thoughts that protected me from actions that may have led to humiliation; thoughts based on a belief that I wasn't capable of many things, not because "I" was incapable, but because my CFS had made me so.

With CFS, I grew accustomed to an internalized life as a hermit. I lived out much of life within the mind—quiet solace. I rarely shared the pain or the inspiration that came from a place of illness. Instead, I found company in the words I wrote on paper, in books I read about health, or in a drawing that expressed some part of my "other" world. CFS was a time of solitude and introspection—the long hibernation before the spring of reemergence.

Now it is springtime both symbolically and in reality. As

the trees flower with blossoms of fragrant pinks, maroons, and yellows, I spring to life with an energy I barely remember. CFS no longer rules; I think I have recovered. But being recovered physically is only part of the picture. I still live out CFS patterns in my mind. I still doubt my capabilities and wonder about my strength. When I find myself getting tired after a busy day, I get scared.

Fatigue still visits on occasion, and with it are reminders of CFS. I find myself deathly afraid at such times, wondering: *Is this remission? Am I really over chronic fatigue? Have I just talked myself into believing that I am in recovery?* As a whirlwind of insecurity spins in my mind, I try to redirect my thoughts.

Like CFS, recovery is also a teacher. Just as CFS is a process rather than an event, so is recovery. One doesn't wake up one day having forgotten all the days before. CFS doesn't disappear in an instant; its presence grows fainter and fainter, while health grows stronger, still stronger. As health improves, CFS beliefs and ways of being are continually tested, and questions emerge. *Do you really think you can do that? What if you get tired or can't remember what to say? What if someone asks you an important question and your mind draws a blank? What if you agree to a com mitment, but find yourself exhausted that day? What if you find yourself getting lost on your way there?* These questions (and others) challenge the newly recovered CFSer. Questions that once protected you from putting yourself in danger or causing you humiliation, now only serve to shoot holes in your self-esteem. They no longer serve you. *Or, do they?*

From my experience, while such questions may provide security and protect me from risk, they may also prevent me from moving past hurdles that are no longer real.

CFS challenges us to define what is real and what isn't. When the rest of the world equates reality with a daily life filled to the gills with activities and *doing,* CFSers instead see life as a moment-to-moment experience lived in slow motion. *Which of these is real?* That is something we all have to decide for ourselves. *And what do we want; what is healthy?*

I believe our society has gone too far in exaggerating the *doing* aspect of life. And CFS brings us to its polar opposite, *being-ness.* In the recovery stage it's time to bring the pendulum back to center, to that in-between place, where *"doing"* and *"being"* exist harmoniously. Currently, I am struggling to find that place for myself.

As I have grown healthier, my desire to swing into action sometimes has led me to swing too far into activity, later regretting it. However, unlike my pre-CFS days, now I have internal sirens that guide me toward a middle-ground between *"doing"* and *"being."* While I haven't yet managed to maintain that balance, I know that as with all aspects of life, this "in-equilibrium" is also part of the process.

Just as I am learning to find equilibrium/balance with my *doing* and *being* states, I do the same with my thinking.

Slowly, I challenge my old beliefs (ones that question my abilities and thinking capacity), and I replace them with new ones.

Unfortunately, many of us want to gauge what works based on our experience. For the CFSer, this is not a reliable measuring stick as our recent past is not a healthy one. Having walked the long CFS path, I am no longer who I was prior to setting out on my CFS journey. Now, I must re-decide who I am. As so eloquently put in *Conversations With God*, book one: *Life is not a process of discovery, but a process of creation.* Without CFS, I would never have experienced the truth of such wise words.

I imagine that many of you have reached this chapter hoping for the perfect happy ending where I recover and that's the end. *Ah, yes, that's that and everything goes back to normal,* you may be thinking. We all like to believe that there is some place to go and once we arrive "there," all the work is done—it's all down hill from here at 101 Easy Street.

The truth is recovery from CFS is not that simple; it's not that life must be a constant struggle either. Rather, it's just that there simply isn't any "there" to get to. Once healed from CFS' bodily symptoms, you will have to heal the CFS mentality. You may find yourself on occasion returning to a busier-than-ever-before lifestyle only to watch yourself get caught up in the whirlwind, then have your mind demand that you pull back. *What did CFS teach you?* Remember: *life is not about what you're "doing;" it's about what you are "being."*

You can "be" anything in the face of action or inaction. Remember Sage, my loving cat; to Sage, life was just about lying around, eating, and sleeping. Yet, at the same time, she also embodied trust, love, acceptance, and patience. She did not "do" much, but her "being" or essence radiated love.

Recently, I took on a job as a research assistant. It seemed easy enough. I actually thought it would be fun and not take a lot of time. Concurrently, I felt like I was finally reentering the "working world," having also started teaching an ESL (English as a Second Language) class. It felt good after a decade of being "away."

Since then, however, as I spend my days working from morning till evening, I find myself separated from my spirit. I feel scattered to the wind, as if I were being blown in ten different directions at the same time. I love what I am doing, but in the act of doing them, I do not love them. Instead, I look outside my car window and gaze longingly at the blooming trees; part of me wants to just return to my lovely yard, sit in my favorite pink chair, and drink up the beautiful change of seasons. I hear myself thinking things like, "I've got to stop this; it's too much; if only I could just sit, just for a bit."

Even as such thoughts leave my mind, I hear another part of me say, "Gretchen, you've got to stop thinking like this or you're going to put yourself right back where you were." And, that, my friends, is how it happens; we get CFS when we send countless thoughts of defeat, spinning, spinning in our minds. With our thoughts and actions, we convey to our bodies what our soul has long since known to be true. Our souls have yearned for some way out of this mess we call our lives. Now that we recognize the pattern and have experienced both the pain and the beauty of CFS, perhaps we can redirect ourselves when we find our thoughts leading us astray.

Know that illness is no longer a necessity to provide you with the lifestyle you want. You no longer need illness to give you an excuse *not* to do something or to inspire change in your life. You no longer need CFS to help you see what is important and what is frivolous.

GEMS

You know that you have reached a crossroads when you reach the time of "reemergence" and now emerge from your past life of fatigue to revisit the world of society and "doing."

Much like the illness that keeps each of us inside a very lonely world, this place of transition can be equally lonely.

Being recovered physically is only part of the picture. One still lives out CFS in the mind, doubting capabilities and wondering about one's strength.

30
REPLACING THE TREE:
IT'S GETTING BETTER

I've got to admit it's getting better, it's getting better all the time.

The Beatles

"I've got to admit it's getting better, getting better all the time." Lying in bed trying to sleep, trying to make up for lost slumber, the Beatles sing, "It's Getting Better," and television's Ally McBeal waves her arms and shakes her head to the tune of my joyful song of healing—all in my head, anyway. I am so much healthier. Years have passed since I wrote most of this book, and CFS has changed my life. I now feel so much healthier, so much more alive; I feel like a new person.

Last night, my husband Carl, a friend, and I walked briskly, weaving in and out of throngs of jazz-loving Montrealers on our way back to our hotel. Carl's friend asked me many questions, among them: *how had I healed?*

As words and thoughts flowed, I shared openly and enthusiastically and found myself explaining that Montreal felt strangely unfamiliar to me because, in a sense, I was not the same person this night as I had been just two years prior when we had lived there. At that very moment as I uttered those words, I became aware of how accurate and surprising they were.

Today, unlike my CFS days, I woke up excited to be alive and with the newfound awareness that, yes, I am a different person from two years ago—vastly different! I have changed. I am happy, confident, and healthy (some, if not most of the time, anyway). How I view and experience the world has changed. My biology, as Catherine Myss calls it, is vastly different from its CFS-dominated days, as are my mind, spirit, and lifestyle.

I have struggled through the darkness and am now piercing through the light. While I am still not completely healed physically, in so many other ways, I am healed. And I know the rest will follow shortly. I share my excitement and this news with you because perhaps your healing has yet to come, and you may doubt it will ever arrive. And you must know: healing is possible and inevitable.

Many CFS books discourage us from believing in improvement, because the authors are only looking at CFS as a physical illness to be cured. They see improvement as being limited to physical wellness and the omission of symptoms. Certainly wellness may express itself through a healthy body, but wellness also comes via other channels, those of healthy mind, emotions, and spirit.

Healing is a divine, complex process and one that begins invisibly. We never actually see the workings or failures of our cells, we simply experience them through how we feel in our bodies. We also experience that feeling better emotionally makes a huge difference in our feelings about ourselves and about our own wellness.

When we focus our thoughts on love, gratitude, and happiness, we tell our bodies to heal, to work, and be the best they can be. And what's more, you don't need medicine to do this—all you need is yourself! We help ourselves to heal within via our thoughts and emotions.

As we begin to feel better, and the pieces of the CFS puzzle fall into place, the former mystery reveals itself. For every person with CFS, there is a different story, one with unique perceptions, events, struggles, symptoms, and healing paths. For each of us has our own unique journey, unique destiny, and our own unique timeline. Such is life.

What I've read and heard about CFS from others often comes from the one-sided focus of experience. People tend to look from the *"outside-in."* We tend to believe that illness begins and ends in the physical body. This is too limited a view for such a profoundly complex illness, one that comes into our lives at stressful times. I am convinced that there are no coincidences, and CFS is no accident.

From the limited physiological (bodily) perspective of CFS comes rigid ideas about prognosis and treatment. How, if there are no clearly defined causes or treatments, can doctors accurately assess a patient's prognosis? I say, "Make up your own!"

Two years ago, I decided I was tired of being tired all the time. Moreover, I was tired of being depressed. I was very depressed, and I knew I couldn't stay that way. A much desired move to Colorado and a mental conviction that, "It was time," were what I needed to begin my recovery.

Recovery begins in the mind. You must decide you want to be better; you must believe you can be better; and you must accept when you're not. Recovery begins invisibly and internally and manifests physically and externally. When you change your mind or decide to think anew, you shift internally. Internal shifts encourage outward action taking. New action encourages internal mind shifts. From wherever you start, you cannot help but impact the whole of your being: your body, your mind, your emotions, and your spirit.

We are our own best healers, truly. We may receive wonderful help from our supportive loved ones, doctors, or healers, but we ultimately do our own healing. We repair ourselves through the choices we make, the actions we take, and the thoughts we choose to think. That is how we heal.

You will heal. It's truly a miraculous discovery to one day realize that you are indeed a different person, a much happier, stronger person than the one you were during, or even prior to CFS' onset. CFS only appears to weaken us so that we can grow strong again, but this time in a new way. We don't just get ill, knock ourselves down, go to bed for five years, and reemerge unchanged. No, that is not our path at all. This is not the path of CFS—CFS *changes* you.

Initially, you may hate the changes. I did. Initially, you may lose. I did. I lost nearly everything. Consider this: perhaps the loss serves a purpose. Maybe we lose it all to gain the realization that we are much more than we once imagined ourselves to be. Perhaps we lose so that we can start fresh and create ourselves anew. Maybe we were too rigid or controlled. Maybe we feared losing. Maybe just some *thing* or things in our selves, in our lives, needed re-arranging.

Whatever the reasons for our lost selves, we will grow, heal, and emerge stronger, happier, and healthier. *How can we not?* CFS demands it, and your soul requires it.

I have made radical nutritional and lifestyle changes. I no longer regularly eat sugar or drink coffee, and rarely eat processed or packaged foods or drink alcohol. I deliberately decide each day how I wish my day to go, and I express gratitude for all that I am and all that I have. I no longer depend on others to make me feel happy, and no longer rely on feeling physically good to feel at peace. I have a true, practiced faith—a connection to the Divine, and I have let go of many issues and conflicts, continuing to observe, reflect, and transform. Without CFS, I don't believe I would have discovered so many wonderful ways to live inwardly as soon as I did, and am truly grateful for what this illness has helped me see and experience. I am ultimately grateful for the struggles because they led me to incredible insight and awareness.

I hope you, my reader, will see CFS as your opportunity to grow, to change, and to evolve into the person you want to be. It's up to you. This is your *Call*.

GEMS

Recovery begins in the mind. You must decide you want to get better. You must believe you can be better.

We are our own best healers truly. We may receive wonderful help from supportive loved ones, doctors, or healers, but ultimately we do our own healing.

Consider this: perhaps the losses in CFS serve a purpose. Maybe we lose it all to gain realization that we are much more than we once imagined ourselves to be. Perhaps we lose so that we can start fresh and create ourselves anew.

Whatever the reasons for our lost selves, we will grow, heal, and emerge stronger, happier, and healthier. How can we not? CFS demands it, and your soul requires it.

APPENDIX I
BODY BASICS FOR CFSERS

She decided to look at her healing as an adventure, commenting, "I always wanted to go exploring, but I sure as hell never thought it would be inside of me."

Caroline Myss

When you try to understand the "whys" and "whats" of your illness, the value of knowing anatomy and how the body works becomes crystal clear. Since finding a knowledgeable, compassionate doctor can be difficult or at times impossible, each CFSer must (to some degree) become his or her own expert.

It is year nine of my CFS journey. While I spent the bulk of this past year feeling great and healthy, more recently CFS has come knocking back on my door. Despite consulting six or so excellent healers, I still find myself having to make key decisions about what to do for my healing.

Today, for example, I awoke to a "period illness" reminiscent of years gone by. As soon as I arose, I felt a wave of extreme sickness wash over me. First, I began feeling nauseous. Then, my body's temperature swung rapidly between hot and cold. And as the wave poured over me, it washed away my energy, throwing me into a tidal wave of pain, nausea, diarrhea, and cold sweats all at once. Each symptom rolled over the other in what felt like a cascade of never-ending illness.

While the above illness was not new to me, it had been something I longed to forget and believed was history. After identifying and treating my hypothyroidism and progesterone deficiencies, the sickness had disappeared. Until today, that is.

A recent dejà vu with what felt like hypothyroidism, and some new symptoms, sent me searching for my old family doctor. Unfortunately, my timing (like so many times before) was poor. My doctor was on baby leave, and I would have to wait for her return or find another doctor. I now had reached a healing crisis, with my fatigue and insomnia heightened and new symptoms sounding off internal alarms. One day in the kitchen, doubled over with brief, albeit alarming, chest pain, I then and there decided to return to my family doctor.

The point of this tale is to illustrate how your need for a doctor may not always be met with immediacy. Sometimes, when you need healing, there just may be no doctor to turn to. At times like these, your own knowledge will prove invaluable. And when you do finally reach the healer's office, your awareness of your symptoms and knowledge of your body will only help you get the care you deserve.

Our bodies are amazingly complex systems. In this section, I will offer a simplistic introduction to each bodily system, adding pertinent CFS-related information where possible.

Since I am not a doctor, I have consulted with healing practitioners to ensure accuracy. Unfortunately, this section can only serve as an introduction to anatomy. To obtain more information, please consult Marieb's *Essentials of Human Anatomy and Physiology* (or another text), a doctor, the Internet, or take a class. Also, please check my website (callforsoulwork.com) for current information on CFS.

YOUR BODY

Our bodies are simple yet amazing intricate master-pieces. That most every creature on the planet has such a complex anatomy is truly awe-inspiring.

Our bodies are made up of 11 unique systems, each designed for specific purposes. All humans have: a skin system, skeletal system (bones), muscular system (muscles), nervous system (brain, spinal cord), cardiovascular system (heart), endocrine system (glandular, hormone), lymphatic system (immune), respiratory system (breathe), digestive system (food breakdown), urinary system (waste), and reproductive system (sexual).

Now let's consider each system, their key organs and functions. For easy access, I have bolded symptoms and systems that are pertinent to CFSers. The asterisks beside some of the body systems denote ones most affected in CFSers.

Skin System

Simply put, this system is what gives our insides protection.

It includes the outer layer of our body, our **skin**, **hair**, and **nails**—the container for everything else. The skin's main function is to protect our tissues as well as regulate temperature via perspiration.

Sketetal System

The sketetal system acts like a foundation does for a building, giving the body structure and support. Its main supports include the **bones, joints, ligaments,** and **cartilage**. The ligaments and joints act like hinges to support the bones and enable our muscles, legs, and arms, to move. The most precious of our bones is the skull (bone surrounding the brain) because it protects our brain. Blood cells develop inside our bones, where the **minerals, calcium** and **phosphorus**, thrive. When the body needs calcium for the nervous system to send messages, or to ask the muscles to contract, calcium is drawn from the bones then passed into the blood vessels and distributed all over the body—wherever it is needed.

Muscular System

Most people associate muscles with strength, but their primary function is movement. Without the body's muscles we would not be able to move and function in all kinds of creative ways. Due to the muscles in our hands, arms, back, abdomen, and legs and their unique ability to contract (or shorten), our body moves. The muscles in our backs, abdomens, and legs give us the support and the posture we expect. Most of our muscles are attached to bones via tendons and ligaments. Through contraction, the muscles create heat. Two exceptional muscles (frequently thought of as organs) include our life-giving heart and the energizing stomach. These will be elaborated on later.

Muscle fatigue, a symptom common to **CFS** and **fibromyalgia sufferers**, occurs when our muscles can no longer contract. Contraction requires oxygen. When contraction is weak or absent, it may be that the body is oxygen-depleted. This can happen when a muscle is over-used or unable to relax due to a deficiency. When a muscle lacks oxygen, lactic acid builds up inside (causing a burning sensation) and the ATP (a cell's life-energy) declines.

In many **CFSers** and fibromyalgia sufferers, **muscle weakness** and/or pain are common. This may be in part because the muscles are over-contracting and not allowed to rest. When you tense your muscles, you also stop your blood from reaching vital organs and the brain.

Nervous System*

The nervous system, our body's telephone system, enables our bodies to communicate with the outside world and our insides (organs) to communicate with us. While straightforward at first glance, the nervous system is actually a complex system. Acting like our bodies' control system, the nervous system can be deeply impacted by CFS. Whenever we experience depression, have difficulty-concentrating, struggle to make decisions, or feel unable to cope, we may be experiencing an unhealthy nervous system. The nervous system consists of our **brain, spinal cord, nerves,** and **sensory receptors**. Any stimulus we encounter, an alarm, the sun's rays, our child's cry, an unexpected snowstorm, all are communicated to us through our nervous system. Every thought, feeling, and action is transmitted through this system. Its primary function, homeostasis (which maintains the body's balance), is maintained via proper signals. Mental processing, emotional reactions, and the chemical absorption or secretion within the glands/organs are dependent on the nervous system. Additional nervous system responsibilities include maintaining our pulse; facilitating our breathing; providing tension for our muscles; ordering our glands to function; and getting blood to flow throughout our bodies.

The nervous system has two parts, the central nervous system and peripheral. The **central nervous system** is "central" to all its operations, the boss. Together, our brain and spine work as a team receiving incoming information through electrical impulses and communicating information to various glands/organs throughout the body.

The **peripheral nervous system** is exactly that; peripheral, or physically away from the rest of the nervous system. This system consists of spinal and cranial (brain) nerves. As their names imply, the **spinal nerves** relay messages to and from the spinal cord, whereas the **cranial nerves** direct messages to and from the brain. All the nerves (long tubes all over the body) act like telephone lines, connecting and communicating chemical messages mainly between muscles/glands and their receptors. Every muscle and gland is connected to the brain and spine via these tubes.

All communication within our nervous system is conveyed by electrical impulses transmitted by the nerve cells, **neurons**. Each nerve cell's basic structure consists of a cell body and a "tail" extending out from the cell body like an arm. It is these "arms" (dendrites and axons) that transmit messages to and away from the cells. You may think of the "arms" as more like antennae. An important element within every neuron is potassium whereas sodium lives just outside the cells. Sodium, along with other minerals, help our bodies use water wisely.

When we are **stressed**, our involuntary nervous system goes into high gear: our muscles tense, blood vessels constrict (tighten), the adrenal glands release cortisol (hormone), and our hearts beat faster. All of these physical reactions make up our "fight or flight" system and enable our bodies to react to situations of danger. In **some CFSers**, these responses are frequently triggered. Over time, excessive triggering of the "fight or flight" response will exhaust the body, especially the adrenal glands (refer to endocrine system).

Endocrine System*

This is by far the most significant system to the CFSer because it is the one that is most altered throughout the course of illness. I recommend that you get to know your endocrine system intimately. The better you understand this system, the easier it will be for you to make decisions regarding any treatments impacting it. (See illustration at the end of Appendix)

All your body's actions, from simple to complex, are a result of this amazing system. For example, how you sleep is determined by the health of the endocrine system, as is whether or not you can have a baby. The endocrine system is made up of numerous glands (10), seven of which are key to the CFSer, with each playing boss to organs in the body. Within this system, glands release hormones, traveling to organs and instructing them in what to do. Our hormones are incredible chemicals released by the glandular cells into the bodily fluid where they direct organ cells to increase or decrease their levels of various chemicals.

There are seven total endocrine glands scattered throughout the body (each creating hormones to regulate functions). Within our brains live three endocrine glands: the hypothalamus, pituitary, and pineal gland. At the base of your neck sits your thyroid and parathyroid glands. Just below those, in the middle of your chest, lives your thymus and seated atop your kidneys are your two adrenal glands. Below that, in the center and a little to the left, is your pancreas. Finally, in men, there are the testes that regulate the sex hormones, and in women, the sex hormones are mainly secreted by the ovaries (Refer to illustration). Now let's look at each gland and the hormones it secretes.

Hypothalamus

The hypothalamus is the master endocrine gland located behind the frontal lobe of the brain. It is important to both the nervous and endocrine systems. For the nervous system, the hypothalamus regulates body temperature, water balance (sodium/potassium), and your metabolism (the breakdown of proteins, fats, and carbohydrates in food). Many of our emotions are also driven by the hypothalamus. This important gland (through the chemicals it produces and releases) also regulates our thirst and appetite, sexual desire, ability to perceive pain and pleasures.

For the endocrine system, the hypothalamus creates two hormones: oxytocin, uterine contractor and milk release inducer, and anti-diuretic hormone (ADH), an urine inhibitor that tells the kidneys to reabsorb water from urine, thus increasing urine and blood. Also, by exerting control on the pituitary's release of hormones, the hypothalamus (through release of its own hormones) is in command of many of the lower endocrine glands. Working as a team, the hypothalamus, pituitary, and adrenals (HPA axis) communicate regularly through a communication loop of hormones. In **CFSers**, some of the endocrine problems such as hypothyroidism or weakened adrenals may be traced to a hypothalamic dysfunction or some problem with the hypothalamus, pituitary, and adrenals or "HPA axis."

Pineal Gland

The pineal gland is a tiny gland set behind your hypothalamus. Little is known about it except that it makes the "sleep" hormone melatonin, whose job is to regulate our circadian rhythms by determining how we respond to light. Our moods are also affected by melatonin (a derivative of the mood-elevator serotonin). [For more on the melatonin-serotonin relationship, see Ross, (02)]

For some CFSers with sleep disturbances, small doses of melatonin may be recommended. I have personally found melatonin helpful as a short-term solution to insomnia. I would not, however, recommend it long term since it is a hormone and its effects are not well known. Instead, Ross (02) and I recommend 5-HTP (derived from the amino acid tryptophan) because it effectively acts as both a sleep aid and mood elevator.

Pituitary Gland

The pituitary gland is a grape-sized gland with two parts (the anterior and posterior) hanging from the hypothalamus. It is greatly influenced by the hypothalamus, but to many lower endocrine glands, the pituitary plays boss. Fundamental to how the endocrine system functions, the pituitary gives orders, via hormones (made up of proteins called peptides), to the lower glands (telling them to increase or decrease certain chemicals). Through a negative feedback loop, the pituitary hormones travel to lower endocrine glands calling each to, in turn, release their own hormones. When hormone levels are too low, the pituitary excretes more of its own hormone to induce the gland to increase its hormone production. When a gland secretes adequate or excessive amounts of its own hormone, it sends a message back to the pituitary telling it so. Thus, the pituitary and the lower endocrine glands work together in a loop of chemical communication.

There are **six pituitary hormones** including growth hormone, prolactin, **FSH** (follicle-stimulating hormone), **LH** (luteinizing hormone), TH or **TSH** (thyroid-stimulating hormone), and **ACTH**. Four of these hormones are sent from the pituitary to lower endocrine glands (these we will consider here).

One of the four hormones released by the pituitary is **LH**, a **female hormone** that tells an ovary (around day 13-14 of the menstrual cycle) when to release an egg (ovulation). In addition, LH encourages the "pre-egg" (or follicle) to produce the female sex hormones, progesterone and estrogen. In males, LH causes the testes to produce testosterone, the primary male sex hormone.

For all females, **progesterone and estrogen** levels are integral to how we feel, experience our periods, and cope with stress. Less influential, but affecting our sex drive, are low levels of testosterone.

In the **female CFSer**, progesterone and estrogen, may fall out of balance. Because progesterone and estrogen fluctuate in response to how other endocrine glands function, the health of the entire endocrine system is vital to the CFSer.

Many hormones and chemicals in the body work together in pairs or groups. Maintaining the proper balance of these pairs of hormones (progesterone/estrogen) or chemicals (potassium/ sodium) is one way the body stays healthy. When there is too little progesterone, for example, estrogen increases, growing out of balance. **Too little progesterone** can cause many uncomfortable symptoms: PMS, cramps, moodiness, inexplicable crying around menses, and abdominal bloating; and too much estrogen can be a serious health risk (more on this in the reproductive system section).

If you experience any of the above symptoms, you

may want to ask your doctor about getting a hormonal test, preferably a panel that measures all estrogens (there are 3) and progesterone levels. A very good test is available from Great Smokies Lab (check Resources).

The second endocrine hormone released by the pituitary is **FSH**, a female hormone. In females, FSH, or follicle-stimulating hormone, does exactly what it sounds like: it stimulates the follicle (what will become an egg) to grow and produce estrogen. This occurs during the first half of menstruation, around day 1-10 of the cycle.

The pituitary's third endocrine hormone is TH or **TSH** (thyrotropic or thyroid-stimulating hormone). TSH tells the thyroid to release more of its own hormone, **thyroxine or T4**. Both TSH and T4 levels are very important to the CFSer as you will see in the thyroid section.

The pituitary's fourth endocrine hormone is **ACTH**. This is a very important hormone because it controls the adrenal glands and their release of **cortisol, adrenaline, and nora-drenalin**. These hormones are very important to the CFSer and will be elaborated on in the adrenal section.

Thymus

Just below the thyroid, in the center of the chest, sits the thymus whose only known function within the endocrine system is the production of the hormone thymosin. To the immune system, however, the thymus controls many immune cells (T cells), and protects the body from invaders by attacking any molecules the body does not recognize.

The thymus is especially important to a child's immune

system as well as the development and storage of white blood immune cells called T-lymphocytes.

Thyroid*

This is one of the most important glands to the CFSer because of its role in our energy. The thyroid's main job is to keep the body running efficiently via its metabolism of glucose (how energy is converted and used), as well as helping tissue development in our nervous and reproductive systems.

Like wings of a butterfly, the two parts of the thyroid wrap around the trachea (windpipe) in the lower part of the neck, with two parathyroid glands decorating each wing (for a total of 4). The health of the thyroid is determined by the amount of the hormone, **thyroxine (T4)**, produced. The pituitary, master endocrine gland, uses its own **TSH** to order the thyroid to make T4. The "T" in T4, stands for the amino acid tyrosine and is combined with 4 molecules of iodine. Once produced, T4 is then converted into T3. This secondary hormone, T3, while making up less than one tenth of the active hormone, exerts greater impact through its efficiency and speed.

Many **CFSers** experience the effects of an inadequate balance between TSH (from the pituitary), T4 and T3. When the thyroid fails to produce enough T4 or T3, it becomes sluggish, signaling **hypothyroidism**. When you feel like you are moving through quicksand, and wake up feeling exhausted; when your muscles are weak and your mind fails you, this could be hypothyroidism. Other common symptoms include low body temperature, cold hands and feet, dry skin, dry and brittle nails and hair.

If you suspect **hypothyroidism**, ask your doctor to test your TSH and free T3 levels or TSH and T4. This way, the doctor can identify the source of the problem, whether it's thyroid or pituitary-related. If you have hypothyroidism, most doctors will want to give you either synthetic or natural thyroid hormone or if you visit a naturopath, you may be given an animal-derived extract made from cow or pig thyroid.

Traditional hormone treatment is fast and can be very effective. The unfortunate side, however, is you may be on the hormone for life. On the other hand, it may be possible to treat or supplement your hormone treatment with Chinese medicine using acupuncture and herbs, or a combination of iodine and tyrosine (or one or the other). Other contributing factors to be aware of are thyroid inhibitors that include fluoride, chlorine, and even soy.

I spent several years on natural thyroid hormones (first Westhroid then Biothroid), both hormones from pigs. While on these hormones I felt good even though I was not symptom-free. At the time, I also had low progesterone and applied progesterone cream daily. Over several years, I brought my thyroid and progesterone levels back into balance by using these treatments, only to have to re-address this imbalance when I went off them.

More recently, I have been getting acupuncture treatments in conjunction with a daily dose of kelp (for iodine) and tyrosine. I have eliminated thyroid inhibitors by filtering the fluoride and chlorine out of my water, and have decreased my soy intake*. Through this regime, over a few months, I have brought my thyroid back into balance and am no longer experiencing the symptoms of lethargy and sluggishness characteristic of hypothyroidism!

In my experience with healers and readings, I've noticed that the common response to hypothyroidism is a hormone prescription. The problem here, in my opinion, is this is a band-aid approach, because it simply gives the thyroid the hormone it is not producing, but does nothing to address the underlying cause of low hormone. I personally prefer to go after the cause, rather than merely treat the symptoms.

In the case of hypothyroidism, there are many factors that could disable the thyroid. (And there are probably other factors in addition to what I mention here.) I have recently noticed just how epidemic hypothyroidism is, and suspect that there may be environmental reasons for this; it would be interesting to know. What is known is that many substances act as thyroid-inhibitors. For example, people exposed to thyroid inhibitors on a regular basis could be adversely affected. For instance, a patient whose tap water is chlorinated, or someone who swims daily in a chlo-

---

* Soy is a controversial subject these days. Many health magazines and holistic health practitioners tout its benefits: healthy protein, low fat, and plentiful phytoestrogens. These phytoestrogens, however, are the culprit: they are either praised for their benefits (especially to pre- and menopausal women), or condemned for those same estrogenic effects. Personally I believe there may be harm in large consumption (several meals a day) because of a correlation I saw between my "night sweats" and high soy consumption.

rinated pool, or someone who eats soy several times a day—all are at risk. Any of these, or a combination thereof, depending upon a person's sensitivity level, could affect one's thyroid hormone levels, therefore perhaps these factors could be considered before adopting a thyroid treatment. I recommend Ross' *Mood Cures* for more information on the thyroid (as well as the whole endocrine system). It does a good job addressing the thyroid—much better than some books dedicated to the subject, and has a lot of invaluable health and mental health information, as well.

Another hormone created by the thyroid is calcitonin. Its role is to lower the levels of **calcium** in the bloodstream by sending the calcium back inside the bones. On the surface of the thyroid's wings, sit four **parathyroid glands**. They secrete PTH, parathyroid hormone, the key regulator of calcium in the blood. **PTH** and **calcitonin** work together in a negative feedback loop to manage adequate blood calcium levels. When blood calcium levels drop to a certain level, the parathyroids release PTH which tells the bones to break down their structure to create more calcium.

The Pancreas

The pancreas, situated in the abdomen on the left side, has the important role of sugar metabolism. Within the endocrine system, the **islets of Langerhans**, tiny endocrine glands dispersed throughout the pancreas, control **insulin** and **glucagon** levels. Working as a team in a feedback loop, insulin and glucagon orchestrate blood glucose levels.

Insulin is a very important hormone. **Sugar-diseases**, (unfortunately increasingly common in our culture) always point back to some problem with insulin-production or its utilization. Diabetes, hypoglycemia, insulin-resistance, and syndrome-X are the new millennium diseases affecting insulin and the pancreas, and likely attributed to our sugar-laden diets.

When we eat sugar, or foods that break down into sugars, our islets of Langerhans (in the pancreas) get busy by rushing insulin into the blood. There, insulin acts like a train delivering glucose to cells. Once inside the cells, glucose is either burned up as energy and converted to glycogen or is converted to fat.

While many hormones have the ability to increase sugar levels, only insulin can lower glucose levels. When sugar or simple carbohydrates are consumed too often, insulin levels are raised so quickly that the pancreas can't keep up. Eventually, the pancreas burns out and insulin response weakens causing "insulin resistance," or worse; if insulin production is jeopardized, diabetes results.

For years, I have experienced **hypoglycemia**. When going too long without food, or when eating too much sugar, I would suffer from weakness, trembling, shaking, irritability, and sometimes headaches. Being aware of this sensitivity, I am careful with my diet (avoiding sugar most of the time, or making sure it is balanced with protein and fat). I also make sure that I eat regularly.

The key to helping your body digest sugar efficiently

is to balance it with fats and proteins to slow down the speed of sugar metabolism. Some people find that taking chromium picolinate or the amino acid L-glutamine reduces sugar craving and crashing. Ross (02) has a lot to say on this.

If you are hypoglycemic, you may want to adjust your diet according to Pavvo (77): 1) eliminate all forms of sugar, 2) replace refined foods with whole grains, 3) decrease or eliminate caffeine, 4) eliminate alcohol and tobacco, and 5) eat moderate amounts of salt.

Two years ago, after regaining ten pounds I had lost, and noticing that most of it had settled on my tummy rather than all-over (my usual pattern), I shared this with my doctor. Also knowing that I still occasionally suffered from anxiety, poor concentration, and intermittent depressed moods (all symptoms of insulin-resistance), my doctor suggested I get tested for insulin-resistance.

After testing positive for **insulin-resistance**, for a month I adopted a special diet (low carbs, good fats, lots of vegetables and fruits, and healthy proteins) and took a "medical food" called "Glycem-X" (by Metagenics). I also began working out at Curves three times per week. Within a month, I had lost the weight, was feeling more energetic, and had improved my insulin response!

Insulin-resistance is characterized by weight gain in the belly, fluid retention, and high cholesterol and blood pressure. While I have never experienced most of these symptoms, I still tested positive. This condition (if untreated) sounds off an alarm, because over time it could lead to syndrome-X, diabetes, heart attack and stroke.

Adrenal Glands*

Every body has two adrenal glands, each that sit atop a kidney and are embedded deep in the abdomen below the ribcage. The adrenals are made up of two distinct parts, the cortex and the medulla. Like other endocrine glands, they communicate directly with the pituitary through a feedback loop. The cortex makes three groups of steroid hormones: **mineralocorticoids, glucocorticords,** and **androgens,** or sex hormones.

The first of these hormones: mineralocorticoids, made on the outer layer of the cortex, are involved in, you guessed it—regulating the mineral and salt content in the blood (sodium, potassium, magnesium). Each of these three minerals talk to the kidneys, letting them decide whether to reabsorb the minerals, or flush them out through the urine—this choice determines **blood pressure levels**. Hoffman, (93)

The **glucocorticoids** (made by the cortex) are a fancy name for the two important hormones, **cortisol** and **DHEA.** Cortisol, (the better understood of the two) helps the body respond to prolonged stress and reduces inflammation and pain. It also plays a role in numerous conditions including asthma, arthritis, and lupus.

DHEA, on the other hand, remains more mysterious, yet is known as a key player in good health. Evidence suggests it contributes to strong energy levels. Blood tests can help doctors assess if either DHEA or cortisol are low. For the

CFSer, the adrenals (and these hormones) frequently play a role in fatigue.

For anyone who experiences pain, severe stress, hypoglycemia, or PMS, these hormone levels may be especially important. While adrenal glands are important to everyone, they are especially significant to **CFSers**. Many CFSers find that much of their fatigue can be traced to **weak adrenals,** rooted in an imbalance in cortisol or DHEA. To identify if you have weakened adrenals, ask yourself: *Do I have difficulty coping with stress? Do I feel like my resist - ances are down? Am I excessively thirsty? Is my endurance not what it used to be or should be?* If you answer "yes" to any or all of these questions, you *may* have a weakness.

People with weakened adrenals lack physical endurance and struggle with exercise; they may have low blood sugar (hypoglycemia), low blood pressure, and low body temperature. Energy levels may feel very limited and chronic lethargy is common. Hoffman, (93)

In addition to the cortex's production of minerals, cortisol and DHEA, it also makes the androgens, testosterone and female estrogens. (These will be discussed further in the "Reproductive System" section.)

The second part of the adrenals, the medulla, helps your body respond to stressful situations through its release of the hormones, epinephrine and adrenaline. When you feel overwhelmed, frightened, or stressed, your neurons tell the medulla when to release **epinephrine** and **norepinephrine (adrenaline)** to ignite the "fight or flight" response; this increases your heart rate, blood, and blood glucose levels giving you herculean energy. It also boosts the lungs and oxygen levels as well.

If you are stressed too often, your body will become exhausted (and undergo all of the physical responses above)—as well as exhaust your adrenals. Hoffman, (93) Much of the fatigue of the CFSer is rooted in exhausted adrenals, and, to heal, reducing the stress load and strengthening the adrenals is vital.

The Cardiovascular System

The cardiovascular system is a life-giving intricate pathway with its chief, the heart, connected to countless tubes, large and small (called arteries and veins). These weave this way and that inside of the body. Each tube carries blood in one direction, to (veins) and away from (arteries) the heart, as well as to and from the organs and glands, in what is called "circulation."

The heart (most important muscle in the body), is a fist-sized organ seated deep in our upper chest between the lungs, a little to the left. A master blood "pumper," the heart, like all muscles, alternates between contraction and relaxation, both pumping blood out and drawing it in.

To pump our blood throughout the body, the heart relies on many large tubes, arteries and veins, and smaller tubes, arterioles and venules, with the capillaries creating webs of the smallest tubes. The further away from the heart the blood is carried, the smaller the tubes become. As blood travels to the lungs, oxygen and nutrients are picked up and at the same time, carbon dioxide is released.

We all know how vital blood pressure is to our health; if too high, it's a heart-hazard and if too low, we grow weak. Blood pressure measures the force of the blood against the vessel walls. The power of this force is what ensures that blood gets to where we need it the most. From the heart, the blood is pushed with greatest force into the largest arteries then travels into the arterioles, capillaries, venules, and veins.

In the **CFSer, low blood pressure** is common. Because it is the constancy of blood flow that delivers oxygen to the muscles and brain, it makes sense that if one has too little blood flow, there is too little oxygen and muscle weakness, fatigue, and poor concentration ensue. While there are many possible causes of low blood pressure, blood pressure on the lower side of normal is considered healthy and the sign of a healthy heart.

The Lymphatic System*

Like the cardiovascular system, which moves fluid (blood) throughout a pathway, the lymph system also moves fluid by way of a system of tubes. The lymphatic system is a quiet, yet important circulatory system made up of a huge highway system of interwoven lymphatic vessels, nodes, organs, and tissues. Its main role is to clean out and drain fluid via T and B cells before the lymph reenters the blood.

Like the cardiovascular system, the lymphatic system is also a transport system with many tubes, however, instead of transporting blood, lymph is its cargo. **Lymph** is made up of water and dissolved proteins. All lymph travels from the venous sites (from smaller tubes at the body's extremities) throughout the body and returns to the heart. On its journey, thousands of nodes (most of which are located around the groin, armpits, neck, and the middle of the waist) filter the lymph.

The powerful lymph nodes marshal our immune systems to protect us from incoming toxins (pesticides, herbicides, chemicals) and foreign molecules (bacteria and viruses) with their fighter lymphocyte cells (B cells). Inside each node, **macrophages** stand alert, ready to consume nasty bacteria or viruses.

Other key immune system players include the spleen, thymus, tonsils, and the Peyer's patches in the intestine. Our spleen sits inside to the left of the abdomen, acting as a filter, cleaning the blood and killing weak red blood cells—what remains is sent off to the liver. For the lymphatic system, the spleen acts as a blood supply tank as well as the creator of fighter T-cells.

Because the **CSFer** may suffer from infections and other illnesses during CFS, it can be helpful to know about the lymphatic system and how it feels when there is an infection. When the nodes are hard at work, they grow and inflame. This swelling causes tenderness, particularly in the large node areas around the groin, navel, neck, and armpits.

The Respiratory System

Without the respiratory system you would go air-free and die. Like the air filter in your car, your lungs clean out unwanted particles from the air before it flows to where it is needed. You take in life-giving oxygen on the in-breath, and get rid of unwanted carbon dioxide on the out-breath. The nose, throat (made up of the pharynx, larynx, and trachea), and lungs all work in unison in this oxygen/carbon dioxide exchange. Through our nose or mouth, we inhale oxygen bringing it deep into our lungs, and through our throats, we exhale carbon dioxide in the reverse direction.

The Digestive System*

The digestive system acts like the fuel system in a car. To be energy-full, we must ingest fuel in the form of food. Just as burned gas creates exhaust, digested food becomes waste. The digestive system is a food and waste system beginning with our mouth (where we put food in) and ending with our anus (where our bowels come out). Making up this important system are the mouth, esophagus (food tube in the throat), stomach, small and large intestines, and anus (rectum). As we digest, food is broken down into its chemical elements. The process begins in the mouth where we chew, and moves through the throat (esophagus), to the stomach, and on to the intestines. Our stomach, liver, pancreas, and intestines all play roles in the breakdown, absorption, and release of waste.

Once our food is swallowed, it passes through the **esophagus**, traveling to the **stomach** where gastric juice (secreted by glands) eats away at it. Next, the **liver** produces a substance called bile, which passes into the small intestine where it emulsifies the fats, breaking large fat molecules down into smaller ones. At the same time the liver does its job, the **pancreas** secretes enzymes that, like the liver's bile, enter into the small intestine.

Of the two intestines, small and large, the **small intestine** does the bulk of food digesting via its enzymes and bile. The large intestine, chief waste manager, dries out the indigestible particles by extracting the water and passing the remaining waste out the rectum as feces.

To the **CFSer**, the digestive process is often disturbed. Constipation tends to be the most common symptom because of a slowed metabolism resulting from decreased activity, disturbed sleep, or hypothyroidism. However, diarrhea, abdominal bloating, and gas can also occur. Many of these complaints can be traced to an imbalance in intestinal flora (healthy internal bacteria living in the intestine walls), or caused by yeast overgrowth (candida albicans or "Candida"). Other times, flora imbalances are attributed to food allergies, nutritional deficiencies, or parasites.

What you eat significantly impacts your intestine. It may be possible to avoid the above discomforts simply by improving the diet. You may wish to test for these conditions (refer to Resources: *Tests to Consider*). Most of all, make sure you get a healthy dose of fiber in the form of fresh fruits, vegetables, legumes, and whole grains.

One way to assess your digestion is to notice how often you have bowel movements and whether they are well formed and not too smelly. Extreme smells, extra soft or firm bowels, or bowel movements less than once a day can all be signals to pay attention to, and may signal one or more of the conditions above.

The Urinary System

Like our digestive system, which takes some stuff in while simultaneously removing certain molecules, our urinary system does the same. It is especially important to us because it allows our bodies to get rid of what we don't need. The urinary system is comprised of two kidneys, ureters, bladder, and the urethra. From each kidney, tubes called "ureters," connect to our bladder where our urine is stored. When urine is ready to pass, it flows from the kidneys through the ureters to the bladder where it passes through the urethra outside the body. The purpose of this system is to flush out nitrogen-containing wastes, maintain the body's water/salt balance, and regulate the acidity (PH) of the blood.

The Reproductive Systems

The **female reproductive system**, between the belly button and groin, consists of the vagina, uterus, fallopian tubes, ovaries, and eggs. To create life, an egg originating inside the ovary as a follicle, travels to the fallopian tube where the sperm will fertilize it.

There are two ovaries (egg sacs) located at the top of each fallopian tube. These house the follicles which will develop into an egg and break free and travel to the fallopian tubes during ovulation. The ovaries produce the hormone progesterone as well as three types of estrogen. At puberty, the pituitary's LH and FSH kick the ovary's hormone production into gear. Estrogens are required to maintain a pregnancy and stimulate the breasts to make milk. Progesterone, along with estrogen, is responsible for the menstrual cycle.

In the **male**, the pituitary uses LH to trigger the testes to produce testosterone as well as sperm. Testosterone is responsible for a man's development of facial hair, heavy bones and muscles, sex drive, and lowering of voice. Once mature, a male adult needs testosterone for sperm production.

The Hormones

In both men and women the reproductive/hormonal system is all about life, making life that is. It is also about sensuality, sexuality, and expressing feelings through our bodies. Sex hormones influence many endocrine glands, some organs, feelings, how we cope with stress (partnering with the adrenals in "fight or flight"; they also impact the thyroid), and even our state of mind.

Female Hormones

For women, the most influential female hormones are **progesterone** and **estrogen** (estradiol, estrone, estriol). Though a complex system, here we will keep it simple. Both progesterone and the estrogens are released in response to the pituitary's LH and FSH. Working as partners in a hormonal dance, progesterone and estrogen play important roles in a woman's health and fertility.

Progesterone means "pro-pregnancy" and is released

during the second half of the menstrual cycle from around the 14th to the 28th day, surging around day 14. This hormone is very important not only to the development of a baby, but to every woman. While progesterone's main role is to ensure pregnancy (making 30 times more in the last three months) as well as birthing a healthy baby, it also partners in the production of three estrogens, testosterone, and cortisol.

Mood-wise, progesterone functions like an **antidepressant** and helps the thyroid to function. It aids the body in **fat-use** and **blood clotting**. Progesterone also plays a role in maintaining oxygen supply and protects our bodies from endometrial and breast cancer.

Despite progesterone's significance, women's bodies make and use estrogen far more. Estrogen helps ensure a healthy vagina by strengthening its lining and cleaning it with secretions. It is also responsible for all the bodily changes a girl goes through from puberty to womanhood including breast and uterine development, and pubic and underarm hair growth. Most estrogen is made in the ovaries, with some derived from fat cells and the adrenals. Neil and Holford, (99)

Male Reproductive System

The pituitary impacts not only the ovaries, but it also releases hormones in males that stimulate the release of the male hormone, testosterone. When a boy's body requires testosterone, the pituitary goes to work, releasing LH. To make a boy into a man, testosterone levels rise, causing the voice pitch to fall, body hair, bone and muscle growth, and the development of sperm inside the testes.

For most men, testosterone levels remain high throughout much of adulthood, ensuring adequate, healthy sperm. For some men, however exposures to environmental toxins, or drugs such as antibiotics, radiation, lead, pesticides, alcohol, or drugs, can hurt sperm and testosterone production. Marieb, (94)

Women and "Estrogen Dominance"

Progesterone and estrogen levels fluctuate regularly throughout a woman's menstrual cycle and lifetime. Like teammates, the two hormones work together to ensure the health of a woman. According to Neil & Holford (99), when the ratio of progesterone to estrogen is altered, with progesterone decreasing or estrogen growing in excess, estrogen dominance occurs.

Once a woman stops ovulating, her progesterone production decreases and the relative amount of estrogen remains high. When the progesterone levels fall, in an effort to tell the ovarian follicles to create more progesterone, the pituitary releases more FSH and LH. When ovulation stops completely, progesterone gradually declines, making the FSH and LH that's already in circulation increase the body's estrogen, and unwanted symptoms associated with "estrogen dominance" soon follow.

Estrogen dominance is a modern-day problem exacerbated by modern day chemicals. According to British nutritionists, Kate Neil and Patrick Holford, society's use of chemicals since WWII has greatly increased, and with them there has been a surge in the incidence of hormone-related diseases. They believe there is a strong correlation between the two. In their book, *Balancing Hormones Naturally*, they describe how many of the chemicals in the environment, (in our food and drugs) are causing hormonal damage, leading to a increase in hormone-related diseases (including cancers).

According to Neil & Holford (99), today, there are over 100,000 synthetic chemicals in circulation, with 15,000 (PCB's) known to have hormone-disturbing effects. At the same time, hormone-related diseases and cancers have risen substantially. As our society has progressed, our use of chemicals has skyrocketed, and we now are exposed to chemicals through our foods, soil, air, water, packages, plastics, and pharmaceuticals. Many of the chemicals used to produce food (pesticides), make cleaning and building products, cosmetics, plastics, and drugs act as **xenoestrogens** in the body, meaning they are absorbed by the body's estrogen sites as estrogen. However, their messages to our reproductive systems do not replicate that of our natural estrogen. Unfortunately, we are all "guinea pigs" in this experiment called modern society, because we don't truly know their impact on the body. What we do know (based on studies of wild animals exposed to these chemicals) is they are harmful and appear to be linked to numerous symptoms and reproductive ailments.

Alarmingly, the chemicals we expose ourselves to may be especially concentrated in the foods we eat. Take farm animals for example. Our farm animals live in giant, crammed warehouses and eat, pesticide-laden, antiobiotic-filled feed. Billions of these abused animals eat hormones in their feed, given solely to fatten them and increase growth rate. When farm animals eat the tainted feed, they accumulate the pesticides, antibiotics, and hormones in their fat, and in turn expose consumers to pesticides, antibiotics, and hormones.

Neil & Holford (99) warn: when we combine the xenoestrogenic exposure (from our food, building products, cosmetics, plastics, and drugs) with that of hormone replacement therapy, HRT, or the "pill" (synthetic sex hormones), we increase our hormone-sensitive tissue as well as our risk of hormone-related cancers. Our overall increased exposure to xenoestrogens may cause "estrogen dominance," and lead to symptoms and diseases such as irritability, memory loss, decreased sex drive, water retention, low blood sugar, hypothyroidism, PMS, endometrial and breast cancer.

While xenoestrogens impact the entire planet, it is easy to see their role in CFS considering the above symptoms. As discouraging as it is to realize the extent of environmental toxins everywhere, it is encouraging to know that we can choose our level of exposure (to some extent), as well as provide our bodies with a defense against them. Neil and Holford, (99) make the following suggestions to help you decrease your xenoestrogen exposure: 1) eat organic food to avoid pesticides and herbicides; 2) avoid chlorine and hundreds of other PCB's by filtering your water; 3) decrease or eliminate your consumption of animal fats to avoid xenoestrogens contained in their feed; 4) decrease your plastic use; 5) use only natural detergents (you can buy these in health food stores); 6) never apply pesticides to your garden, and 7) avoid the synthetic hormones, HRT, and the "pill."

Airola, Paavo. *Hypoglycemia: A Better Approach*, Sherwood, OR: Health Plus Publishers, 1996.

Hoffman, Ronald. *Tired all the Time*, New York, NY: Pocket Books, 1993.

Lark, Susan. *Chronic Fatigue and Tiredness: A Self-Help Program*, Los Altos, CA: Westchester Publishing Company, 1993.

Murray, Michael. *Chronic Fatigue Syndrome: How You Can Benefit From Diet, Vitamins, Minerals, Herbs, Exercise and Other Natural Methods*, Rocklin, CA: Prima Publishing, 1994.

Marieb, Elaine, *Essentials of Human Anatomy and Physiology*, fourth edition, Redwood City, CA: The Benjamin/Cummings Publishing Company, Inc., 1994.

Neil, Kate & Holford, Patrick. *Balance Hormones Naturally*, Freedom, CA: Crossing Press, 1999.

Teitelbaum, Jacob. *From Fatigued to Fantastic*, Garden City Park, NY: Avery Publishing Group, 1996.

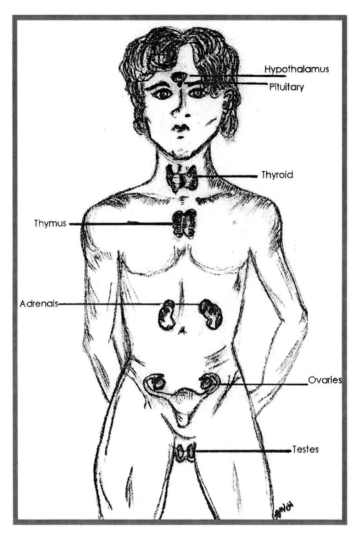

The Endrocrine System
male/female combined

CFS Resources

As of June 2004, there are over a million websites dedicated to CFS underscoring both its pervasiveness and peoples' need for information on the subject. To help you reduce internet-induced headaches, I have included here some helpful, informative websites as well as additional resources.

WEBSITES
The CFIDS Organization
www.cfids.org
I highly recommend becoming a member, as you will receive a journal and regular information on current research, conferences, and events.

CFS is Call For Soulwork *(my website)*
www.callforsoulwork.com
An uplifting and informative website to empower the CFSer.

Fatigue and Fibromyalgia Clinic of Michigan
www.cfids.com

OFFER: Organization for Fatigue and Fibromyalgia Education and Research

www.offerutah.org

The Center for Disease Control

www.cdc.gov

National Institute of Allergy and Infectious Diseases

www.niaid.nih.gov

The American Academy of Nutrition

www.nutritioneducation.com

Immune Support and Chronic Pain Specialists

www.immunesupport.com

Dr. Jacob Teitelbaum
   (doctor specializing in chronic fatigue)

www.endfatigue.com

Dr. Susan Lark
   (information on fatigue and women's health)

www.drlark.com

Dr. Andrew Weil
   (doctor specializing in holistic medicine)

www.drweil.com

Thomas Day Oates, Jr.

(CFSer offering spiritual CFS tapes)

www.healing-peace.com

CFS NETWORK

The CFIDS Association of America

This network publishes two journals, conducts CFS research, provides CFS support and information, and can help you locate support groups.

The CFIDS Association of America

P.O. Box 220398

6827-A Fairview Road

Charlotte, NC 28210

(800) 442-3437

www.cfids.org

ORGANIZATIONS RELATED TO CFS

Food Allergy Network

The Food Allergy & Anaphylaxis Network

11781 Lee Jackson Highway, suite 160

Fairfax, VA 22033

(800) 929-4040

www.foodallergy.org

American Chronic Pain Association Outreach

(916) 632-0922

www.theacpa.org

BLOOD & STOOL TESTING

Great Smokies Diagnostic Lab

63 Zillicoa Street

Asheville, NC 28801-1074

www.gsdl.com

TESTS TO CONSIDER

(Not in order of importance)

Female Hormones

For: PMS, moodiness, fertility

1. Woman's Hormonal Health Assessment: Measures progesterone, estrogens, testosterone, and DHEA (Great Smokies Diagnostic Lab)

Thyroid

Beware: many thyroid imbalances are missed if both tests are not done; many physicians only measure TSH.

1. TSH (Thyroid Stimulating Hormone)
2. Free T3 or T4

Sugar Diseases

For: hypoglycemia, diabetes, insulin-resistance, syndrome X

1. Glucose Tolerance Test (hypoglycemia)
2. Insulin, fasting (hypoglycemia, diabetes, insulin resistance, syndrome X)

Adrenals

1. DHEA
2. Cortisol

Candida (yeast overgrowth)

1. Blood test

Immune, Kidneys, Liver Function

1. CBC (Complete Blood Count)

Food Allergies

1. ELISA blood test: measures immunoglobins G and E's response to large list of foods
2. RAST blood test: measures IgE's response to certain foods
3. Skin Prick Test: measures skin's reaction to foods (administered by needle to forearm)

Environmental Toxins: Heavy Metals

1. Elemental Hair Analysis from Great Smokies Diagnostic Lab: measures key minerals (calcium, magnesium, copper, zinc...), important nutrients (iodine, selenium...), toxic metals (aluminum, arsenic, cadmium, mercury, lead...), as well as sodium, potassium, and phosphorus...
2. Urine Test from Great Smokies Diagnostic Lab: More accurate than the hair test and requires first taking a metal extractor (DSMA, for example) and then collecting urine for 24 hours.

Disease Contributor: Body PH

Tests the body's overall PH. Too much acidity contributes to disease.

1. Purchase a tape from physician to test urine or saliva.

RECOMMENDED READING
CFS BOOKS

Most CFS books focus on the physical-side of this illness emphasising medical information (all except Duff's here): causes, diagnosis, symptomology, and treatment, and many unfortunately read like medical journals.

I found the following books, however, to be extremely helpful and relatively easy-to-digest. This sample represents maybe a tenth of what's out there. And to be quite candid, even these books were often too difficult to assimilate when CFS robbed me of my ability to concentrate. Now, years after their initial purchase, I am reading them again and am truly amazed at the wealth and breadth of information here. I am also surprised by how much what is covered in these books mirrors my experiences in terms of symptoms, treatment, and philosophy.

I am recommending these books to you because I believe they can help you identify the causes of your CFS and give you helpful treatment suggestions. While some are difficult to read, they are well worth their time and effort. Also, each is sensitive to the CFSer and many share personal portraits and fascinating CFSer anecdotes.

While each of these books has so much to offer, even one such book could overwhelm the CFS sufferer with mental challenges. This is why I suggest that you don't follow my lead; do not keep buying. Instead, try picking one or two CFS books that can truly help you. Go to a large bookstore, library, or online and locate one with a hefty CFS section. Browse until you find one that feels "right."

Choosing the "right" book is a lot like choosing the "right" anything. What works for you, will not necessarily work for me, and vice-versa. You must choose. The act of finding a helpful CFS book is a sacred part of the CFS heal - ing journey—much like finding a good doctor. They are hard to find, but when you do find one, the effort proves worth the journey. This, my friend, is all part of the journey, part of knocking down the CFS tree, and part of your Call For Soulwork.

Agombar, Fiona. **Beat Fatigue with Yoga, the Simple Step-by-Step Way to Restore Energy**, Hammersmith, London: Thorsons, 2002.

While Fiona's book is primarily a yoga guide for the CFSer (a very good one at that), it also offers helpful insights into some causes of fatigue, yoga lifestyle (postures, breath, diet), energy and energy channels (chakras), and practical suggestions for re-balancing the mind and body. Her prose is friendly as well as upbeat, and personalized by her own CFS story as well as the stories of others.

Duff, Kat. **The Alchemy of Illness**, New York: Bell Tower, 1993.

Kat Duff weaves ideas poetically in her CFS novel rich in soulwork and insights. I recommend this book to the CFSer with a well mind and a strong desire for validation.

327

Gellman, Lauren, M. & Erica F. Verrillo. **Chronic Fatigue Syndrome: a Treatment Guide**, New York, NY: Saint Martin's Griffin, 1997.

This is a must-have compendium of hundreds of CFS symptoms, ailments, and their suggested treatments. Its dictionary-like coverage includes mainstream medical approaches as well as alternative medical therapies.

Hoffman, Ronald. **Tired All the Time: How to Regain Your Lost Energy**, New York, NY: Pocket Books, 1993.

Like so many other CFS books, this work focuses on the underlying contributors to fatigue, covering a sweeping range of areas: hormones, environmental toxins, sugar-related diseases, allergies, and depression. It is especially unique in its exploration of environmental contributors to CFS and sugar-related illnesses.

Kenny, Timothy. **Living with Chronic Fatigue Syndrome: A Personal Story of the Struggle for Recovery**, New York, NY: Thunder's Mouth Press, 1994.

If you seek a personal story that shares both the struggles of CFS as well as a layperson's perspective on the medical aspects of CFS, than this could be the book for you. Kenny tells about a 5-year struggle to work in broadcasting despite debilitation and brain deterioration. Chronicling his evolution through job loss and denial, Kenny's physical pain is surmounted by the pain he feels in giving up the only identity he knows—that of work.

Lark Susan. **Chronic Fatigue and Tiredness: A Self-Help Program**, Los Altos, CA: Westchester Publishing Company, 1993.

This was my first CFS book and it continues to be one of my favorites. Lark is thorough in her exploration of the causes of fatigue and in suggesting treatment. Using the book's questionnaires tailored to each condition, it's possible to root out which symptoms are attributed to which ailments (an amazing feat for any CFSer). In addressing each condition separately (Candida, hypothyroidism, PMS, and menopause...), specific comprehensive treatment plans are laid out.

Murray, Michael. **Chronic Fatigue Syndrome: How You Can Benefit from Diet, Vitamins, Herbs, Exercise, and other Methods**, Rocklin, CA: Prima Publishing, 1994.

Based on a naturopath's holistic approach to CFS, Murray takes an in-depth look at the possible causes of CFS and tailors treatment plans to address the mind, diet, sup - plements, bodywork, and exercise. This book may be a very helpful addition to your CFS library; however, it also may read overly technical for the foggy-brained CFSer.

Teitelbaum, Jacob. **From Fatigued to Fantastic: a Manual for Moving Beyond Chronic Fatigue and Fibromyalgia**, Garden City, NY: Avery Publishing Group, 1996.

Teitelbaum brings both personal and professional wisdom to CFS (having once had the illness himself, and now working closely with CFS sufferers in his practice as physician). Taking a compassionate approach to CFS, he

329

examines the underlying physical causes of CFS and how they interact together. He considers the roles of hypothy - roidism, Candida, nutritional deficiency, food allergies, and chemical sensitivity, and gives treatment suggestions for each. This book is especially helpful to the health practition - er (it is my family doctor's CFS bible), because of its informa - tion on testing, interpretation, and medical studies. While medically dense, this book is reader-friendly.

For Parents (Children's book)

Nassar, Gretchen Brooks. **What's Wrong with Mommy?** Fort Collins, CO, 2004.

This is a children's picture book (currently without illus - trations) written especially for children aged 6-9 who have a parent with CFS. The book confronts the meaning of CFS in one family.

To order a copy, write to: gretchen@callforsoulwork.com

CFS Book Criteria

To aid your CFS book selection process, I am including a list of key criteria. Under each author's name, you will encounter a list of what is included in each book.

Agombar

Alternative medicine

Author's story

CFSer perspective

Easy-to-read

Yoga program

Duff

Alternative medicine

Author's story

Gellman

Alternative medicine

Anecdotes

Encyclopedic

Easy-to-read

Great resources

Mainstream medicine

Treatments (100's)

Hoffman

Alternative medicine

Anecdotes

Diagnostic questionnaires

Doctor's perspective

Environmental impact

Exercise

Mainstream medicine

Medically-dense

Treatments

Kenny

Anecdotes

Author's Story

CFSer Perspective

Easy-to-Read

Mainstream Medicine

    (From the author's personal perspective)

Lark

Anecdotes

Alternative medicine

Comprehensive treatments

Diagnostic questionnaires

Doctor's perspective

Easy-to-read

Exercise

Mainstream medicine

Recipes

Yoga program

Murray

Alternative medicine

Comprehensive treatment plans

Diagnostic questionnaires

Doctor's perspective

Environmental impact

Exercise

Medically-dense

Mind-body

Recipes

Teitelbaum

Author's story

CFSer perspective

Comprehensive treatment plans

Doctor's perspective

Doctor section

Mainstream medicine

Medically-dense

Questionnaires

Some alternative medicine

RECOMMENDED READING
HEALTH & HEALING BOOKS

Airola, Paavo. **Hypoglycemia: A Better Approach**, Sherwood, OR: Health Plus Publishers, 1996.

Balch, James F. & Phyllis A. **Prescription for Nutritional Healing, A Practical A-Z Reference to Drug-free Remedies Using Vitamins, Minerals, Herbs & Food Supplements**, Garden City Park, NY: Avery Publishing Group, 1997.

Ballentine, Rudolph, **Diet & Nutrition: A Holistic Approach**, Honesdale, PA: Himalayan Press, 1978.

Cousins, Norman. **Anatomy of an Illness**, New York, NY: W.W. Norton, 1979.

Crook, William G. **The Yeast Connection Handbook**, Jackson, TN: Professional Books, Inc., 1997.

Neil, Kate and Patrick Holford. **Balance Hormones Naturally**, Freedom, CA: Crossing Press, 1999.

McIntyre, Anne. **The Complete Woman's Herbal: A Manual of Healing Herbs and Nutrition for Personal Well-Being and Family Care**, New York, NY: Henry Holt Reference Book, 1994.

Myss, Caroline. *Why People Don't Heal and How They Can*,
New York, NY: Three Rivers Press, 1997.

Northrup, Christiane. *Women's Bodies, Women's Wisdom: Creating Physical and Emotional Health and Healing*,
New York, NY: Bantam Books, 1998.

Null, Gary, *Nutrition and the Mind*,
New York, NY: Four Walls Eight Windows, 1995.

Robbins, John. *Diet for a New America: How Food Choices Affect Your Health, Happiness and the Future of Life on Earth*, Wadpole, NH: Stillpoint Publishing, 1987.

Siegel, Bernie. *Peace, Love and Healing: Bodymind Communication & the Path to Self-Healing: an Exploration*,
New York, NY: Harper Perennial, 1989.

Weil, Andrew. *Spontaneous Healing*,
NH: Alfred A. Knopf, 1995.

RECOMMENDED READING
SPIRITUAL BOOKS

Albom, Mitch. **Tuesdays with Morrie**, New York,
   NY: Bantam Doubleday Dell Publishing Group, 1997.

Hay, Louise L. **You Can Heal Your Life**, Carlsbad,
   CA: Hay House, Inc., 1999.

Jampolsky, Gerald G. **Love is Letting Go of Fear**,
   Berkeley, CA: Celestial Arts, 1979.

Matthews, Andrew. **Being Happy**, Los Angeles, CA:
   Price Stern Sloan, 1990.

Millman, Dan. **Way of the Peaceful Warrior, A Book that
   Changes Lives**, Tiburon, CA: H.J. Kramer, Inc., 1980.

Vanzant, Iyanla. **One Day My Soul Just Opened Up**,
   New York, NY: Fireside, 1998.

Walsch, Neale Donald. **Conversations With God: book one**,
   New York, NY: G.P. Putnam's Son, 1995.

Walsch, Neale Donald. **Conversations With God: book two**,
   Charlottesville, VA: Hampton Roads, 1998.

Walsch, Neale Donald. **Conversations With God: book three**, Charlottesville, VA: Hampton Roads, 1998.

Walsch, Neale Donald. **Friendship With God**, New York, NY: G.P. Putnam's Sons, 1999.

About The Author

Gretchen Brooks Nassar Lives in Fort Collins, Colorado with her loving husband, Carl, and two cat companions, Sylvan and Sumu. In May 2001, she completed her MA at Colorado State University in English. For several years, Gretchen taught English to adult immigrants as a volunteer and through her *Living English* business. She also holds a BA in psychology from Sonoma State University. Throughout Gretchen's ten-year journey with CFS, she has studied holistic health (nutrition, herbology,

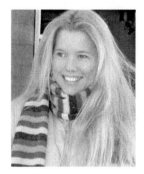

aromatherapy, homeopathy, ayurveda, and attunement). Her role in the community includes that of writer, teacher, and artist, and her life is filled with numerous passions including being an animal advocate and vegetarian.

Gretchen invites readers to share their CFS stories, as well as their reactions to this book. Please e-mail her at *gretchen@callforsoulwork.com*. Also, to get updated CFS information, read CFS related articles, and to see all *Call*

For Soulwork products, go to *www.callforsoulwork.com.*

You can order the following products online at *www.callforsoulwork.com*

- This book: *CFS is a Call For Soulwork*
- The *Call For Soulwork Booklet* (a compilation of quotes from *CFS is a Call For Soulwork*)
- Children's Book: *What's Wrong with Mommy?*
- *Call For Soulwork* bookmarks

CPSIA information can be obtained at www.ICGtesting.com
Printed in the USA
BVOW04s0038241014

372076BV00001BA/44/P